The New Zealand

3am

HANDBOOK

The New Zealand

3am

HANDBOOK

The most commonly asked questions about your child's health

DR WILLIAM FELDMAN

Adapted for New Zealand by the Starship Children's Hospital

First published in New Zealand in 2001 by
TANDEM PRESS
2 Rugby Road
Birkenhead, Auckland
New Zealand
www.tandempress.co.nz

First published in Canada in 1997 by
Key Porter Books Limited

Reprinted 2003 (twice)

ISBN 1 877178 60 8

Cover design and text production by Verso Visual Communications
Text design by Leah Gryfe
Photography by Kirsty Pattinson
Printed in New Zealand by Publishing Press Ltd

Acknowledgements

We would like to thank the team of professionals from the Starship Children's Hospital, the University of Auckland (Injury Prevention Research Centre) and SafeKids who gave their time and expertise to adapt this book for New Zealand. They are:

Rhonda Akroyd
Dr. Richard Aickin
Dr. Shanthi Ameratunga
Dr. Raewyn Gavin
Dr. Cameron Grant
Marina Johnson
Dr. Patrick Kelly
Dr. Alison Leversha
Katherine Lissienko
Helen McCracken
Dr. Jocelyn Neutze
Dr. Ralph Pinnock
Dr. Nikki Turner

General Editor

William Feldman, MD, FRCPC

Co-Authors

Paul Dick, MD, CM, FRCPC

Darcy Fehlings, MD, FRCPC

William Feldman, MD, FRCPC

Marvin Gans, MD, FRCPC

Alan Goldbloom, MD, FRCPC

Saul Greenberg, MD, FRCPC

William Hanley, MD, FRCPC

Robert Hilliard, MD, FRCPC

Moshe Ipp, MBBCh, FRCPC

Sheila Jacobson, MBBCh, FRCPC

David Lloyd, MD, FRCPC

Patricia Parkin, MD, FRCPC

Norman Saunders, MD, FRCPC

Clive Schwartz, MBBCh, FRCPC

Susan Tallett, MBBS, FRCPC

Lionel Weinstein, MD, FRCPC

Contents

Introduction

· ·

The purpose of this book is to provide parents with general information about their children's health, based not just on opinion but on sound scientific evidence. No attempt has been made here to describe every disease and condition that can affect children; instead, this book covers extensively the troublesome aspects of 'normal' behaviours of children such as eating and sleeping problems.

All parents ask themselves 'how' questions – 'How can I protect my child from injuries?'; 'How can I tell if there's something seriously wrong with my child?'; 'How can I improve my child's eating habits?' For answers they often turn to their family doctors or paediatricians, or to books and articles by doctors. They look for answers that are based on years of practical experience.

Although the knowledge gained from practical experience is immensely valuable, it's not the only source – or necessarily the best one – for answers to those 'how' questions. A doctor's conclusions may be affected by the particular population of patients he or she serves, or by his or her own philosophy or expectations. This 'personal' aspect is the reason that hospitals and other medical institutions carry out a broad range of clinical research studies and controlled trials. By eliminating personal bias, and methodically comparing results in large numbers of children, it's possible to say with much more certainty what behaviour is 'normal' and what is not, what treatment 'works' and what does not.

This book is adapted from one written by highly trained paediatricians, and members of the Division of General Pediatrics at the Hospital for Sick Children, in Toronto. This edition was adapted for use in New Zealand by paediatricians at Starship Children's Hospital. We all share an interest in 'evidence-based medicine', medicine based on the science of clinical epidemiology – in other words, based on organised, disciplined research into how children really behave, how we can keep them healthy, and how we can best help them when they are unwell.

Collectively, of course, we have hundreds of years of personal experience in taking care of children, both healthy and sick. But while we are focusing on our individual child patients, we are also asking ourselves more general questions – the same 'how' questions that parents ask – and looking for ways to test procedures and beliefs.

We hope the answers we've found will resolve some of the questions you've been asking yourselves, and will help you through the exciting, exhilarating, and sometimes *exasperating* challenge of raising your children to be the best they can be!

CHAPTER 1

Choosing Your Child's Doctor

● ●

hen young doctors are about to go into practice, they often ask older doctors what they need to do to be successful. For many years the standard answer has been: 'Demonstrate the three A's.' They are, in order of importance, *ability*, *availability*, and *affability*. When you're choosing a doctor for your child, these are three essential qualities to keep in mind. Many families will use the same general practitioner for themselves and their children. If you have moved to a new area you may need to find a new doctor.

Q **What exactly do you mean by 'ability'?**

In *Webster's New World Dictionary*, 'ability' is defined as 'power to do [something]; talent; skill.' The powers, talents, and skills your child's doctor should have can be categorised into four broad areas: prevention, diagnosis, treatment, and rehabilitation.

In the field of *prevention*, your child's doctor should be aware of which preventive measures work and which don't. For example, certain screening tests for newborns are very effective in preventing mental handicap or physical disability, and should be performed on all newborns. 'Well-baby visits' – routine medical checkups when nothing seems to be wrong – provide immunisation and advice that can prevent life-threatening problems later on.

Diagnosis means discovering the root of a problem such as fever, pain, difficult breathing, or disturbing behaviour. The doctor should be skilled at reaching a diagnosis by various means. The first and most important is simply asking the parents (and children, if they are not too young) for a description of the problem: whether it's getting better or worse, what makes it better or worse, how it's affecting the child's (and family's) life. The answers often go a long way towards identifying the cause of the problem. The second means of diagnosis is the physical examination. The third is laboratory tests. In general, the more experienced doctors are in diagnosing and treating the medical problems of children, the less they depend on lab tests. There are, of course, problems that require certain tests or X-rays, but the most able diagnosticians rely heavily on asking questions and on physical exams.

The fourth means of diagnosis is referring the child to another doctor for consultation. Some doctors are so busy seeing large numbers of patients that they don't have time to ask the extra questions or to do the detailed physical examination needed for a diagnosis; they tend to refer too many children to specialists. Other doctors are overly confident of their own abilities, and they may not refer enough children to specialists.

Modern *treatment* has changed dramatically in the last hundred years. In the old days doctors didn't have a lot of effective medications or surgical procedures to offer, so they were much better at diagnosis than at treatment. In the last century, however, we have developed a host of effective treatments, as well as more sophisticated diagnostic tools. However, just as the treatments have become more powerful, so have some of the side-effects become more serious. Therefore, the most able doctors are those who use treatments that have been shown to do more good than harm. Fortunately, modern doctors – and increasingly aware consumers – are asking for proof that a treatment is necessary, and that the outcome is likely to be better than it would have been with no treatment.

Rehabilitation is the fourth critical area of skill. Some problems, like asthma or cerebral palsy, are 'chronic' and can't be cured – we just have to live with them. An able doctor tries to rehabilitate a child with a chronic problem, to enable the child to live with as few limitations as possible. In the case of asthma, medication given when the child is well will usually prevent attacks and allow the child to attend school and play sports. In the case of cerebral palsy, the doctor should know which medical and non-medical specialists can help the child lead as full a life as he or she can.

 ## How much 'availability' should I expect from a doctor?

Children get sick, and parents have anxieties, at all times of the day and night. Most often the experienced parent knows when a problem is a real emergency and the child needs to be seen by a doctor without delay. But parents need time to acquire experience, and they need sources of information. We hope this book will help you determine when it's necessary to call your doctor at 2:00 A.M., or rush to an emergency department; we also hope to give you some advice on what steps you yourself can take to make your child feel better while you're deciding whether to call the doctor.

Nevertheless, most parents, no matter how experienced and knowledgeable they are, will need to get in touch with their doctor sometime because their child has an acute problem. And that's when accessibility becomes crucial. Even during office hours, a very busy doctor may be hard to reach because the telephone is constantly in use. Many doctors get around this by having extra telephone lines, so parents can always get through.

Of course, the big problem with availability comes during nights, weekends, and holidays.

Some general practitioners work with a group of other doctors to form a roster so that one doctor is always available. Many centres have after-hours clinics for urgent problems.

The availability of their doctor gives parents a sense of security, and it's also important for other reasons. A telephone discussion between the parent and a doctor solves the majority of after-hours problems; the doctor gets enough information to decide whether the child needs to be seen at once, and in more than half the calls the decision is that there is no need for a doctor to see the child. This not only saves money for the health-care system, but also spares the family a lot of trouble and lost time. Furthermore, each episode successfully handled with after-hours telephone consultation helps give parents the experience and knowledge they need to become less dependent on the health-care system.

No parent can expect a doctor to be on call 24 hours a day, seven days a week. Years ago many doctors did practise this way, making housecalls, creating a special bond of caring between themselves and the families they served. Although they didn't have many effective treatments to offer, they demonstrated a helping mission that was in itself often therapeutic.Nowadays doctors have many effective treatments to offer, but until fairly recently medical schools concentrated on the curing, not the caring, aspects of being a doctor. That is now changing, as medical educators try to develop an appropriate balance of curing and caring in selecting and educating future doctors.

Most doctors these days practise in on-call groups; this approach enables patients to obtain immediate advice, and doctors to have time for their personal lives.

Why does 'affability' matter in a doctor?

Webster's defines 'affable' as 'easy to speak to; approachable.' We use 'affability' to mean the quality that makes you feel at ease talking with a doctor – confident that you aren't being rushed out, that the doctor really is interested in discussing your concerns. This climate of interest should be apparent in all office staff – the receptionist, nurse, and others in the practice.

There are several ways the doctor and staff can demonstrate their interest and concern. One is the office setting itself. Although it need not be luxurious, it should at least be pleasant and comfortable, particularly the waiting area. There should be interesting, up-to-date reading material for readers of all ages, as well as toys and games for younger children. The most important components of affability, however, are the interpersonal skills of the doctor and staff, and the feeling that you are not being processed on an assembly-line.

The interpersonal skills should include friendliness and the demonstration of a genuine affection for children. Also, the doctor should use language the child understands. Often a child can help in arriving at a diagnosis. For example, if a nine-year-old has recurrent tummy-aches, the doctor may ask the parent if there is any constipation – a common cause of abdominal pain. But the parent may have no idea of the child's bowel habits, and the child may not understand what 'constipation' means. If the doctor asks the child, 'Does your bottom hurt when you poo?' and the answer is yes, the problem may be solved.

This easy communication should exist at all stages of the system. When you telephone for information or an appointment, you should be made to feel that your request is as important to the doctor and staff as it is to you. When you are seeing the doctor with your child, you should be made to feel that you can discuss anything you wish and that the doctor won't consider it frivolous. When a test is being ordered, you should feel free to ask why it's being done and how the results of the test will affect your child's treatment. You should never leave the office with questions you would have liked to ask. In fact, the affable doctor will usually ask if you have any unanswered questions, or anything else you would like to discuss, before you leave.

The best doctors combine ability with availability and affability. Although these are also the doctors with fairly large practices, they usually have excellent time-management skills, and the people in their care don't feel rushed.

···

Finding an able, available, and affable doctor for your child

···

1. Talk to friends, relatives, and neighbours about the doctors who have looked after their children. Ask about the quality of care given, not only by the doctor, but by the nurse and receptionist. Is it easy to get through to the office, or is the line always busy? Are the people friendly? Is the office child-oriented? Does the night and weekend message refer to a walk-in clinic or emergency department, or does it pass your number to an on-call doctor? Get the names and numbers of the three or four doctors who sound best to you.

2. Visit the office of the doctor who ranks highest on your list. In making the appointment, tell the truth: you are looking for a doctor for your child, and you would like to meet the doctor, even though your child is currently healthy, or is not yet born. During your visit, assess the office, the staff, and the general atmosphere. If your own opinion agrees with the 'word of mouth,' you've probably found the right doctor.

Should I look for a paediatrician, or a family doctor?

In some communities there's no choice – the only health-care practitioners available for children are family doctors, who are trained to look after the entire family. The amount of training they have in paediatrics (care of children) varies. Generally, they will have had an average of two months of paediatrics, but many see a lot of children during their training programme. Paediatricians are specialists who have had at least five years of training specifically involving children.

Some paediatricians work in private practice and others in public hospitals and clinics. To see a paediatrician in a public clinic requires a referral from your family doctor.

Another medical professional is the nurse practitioner – a nurse who has extra training in diagnosis and treatment. This profession is fairly new in New Zealand.

CHAPTER 2

Your Child at Birth

● ●

Though the birth of a baby is a wonderful natural event, there is always a small chance of something going wrong. In the past, a significant proportion of infants suffered damage, either from the birth process itself, or from conditions that were present at birth and were not treated.

These days we have a wide selection of tests, treatments, and procedures that can be used before, during, and after delivery to give a newborn the best possible start. But some parents feel that in focusing on medical aspects of birth, hospitals have intruded too far into what is usually an uncomplicated, joyous family event. The trend now is towards maintaining the intimate family connections of birth as far as possible, while still taking precautions and being prepared for the unforeseen.

 Where should babies be born: at home, in hospital, or in a birthing centre?

It's well documented that 85 to 90 percent of deliveries are full-term and uneventful. The remaining 10 to 15 percent involve some sort of complication, but most can be predicted prior to labour, or in the first stage of labour, and appropriate preparations can be made – such as having an obstetrician and a paediatrician/neonatologist (specialist in newborns), present at the delivery. The worrisome cases are those in which the complication doesn't occur until the second stage of labour, when the cervix is fully dilated and delivery is imminent. These late complications include compression or prolapse (early expulsion) of the umbilical cord, premature separation of the placenta, obstructed delivery, and bleeding. Any one of these can reduce the amount of oxygen reaching the baby's brain, which could have serious permanent effects. When one of these complications arises

 16

in hospital, skilled, well-equipped caregivers are on hand to provide immediate help. But if something like this happens in the home, or even in a 'stand alone' birthing centre, there may be significant delay in treating the baby.

If delivery is to be outside a hospital, by a family doctor or midwife, be sure provisions have been made for immediate help if any unforeseen circumstances arise.

What steps are taken once the baby is born?

The nose and mouth of the baby may be cleared of body fluids, the umbilical cord is clamped and cut. The baby may be given to the parents for a little while then moved to a special resuscitation table under a heat lamp and is dried off, to prevent heat loss. There can be serious problems in infants who have been stressed by cold at birth. When the infant is about one minute old, an assessment called an Apgar test is carried out. If the score is below 7, various resuscitative measures are undertaken. These may range from supplying oxygen through a mask to passing a breathing tube down the baby's airway, massaging the heart, using medication to stimulate the heart, and supplying intravenous fluids and drugs. At five minutes of age, another Apgar assessment is carried out, to tell the doctor or midwife if further resuscitative measures and closer observation are needed.

At this point a brief physical examination is carried out by the doctor or midwife in attendance. An identification band is placed around the baby's

Scoring the Apgar test

Sign	Points		
	0	1	2
Colour	pale/blue	pink with blue extremities	pink body
Heart rate	not detected	below 100	over 100
Irritability	no response	grimace	lusty cry
Muscle tone	flaccid	some movement	vigorous
Breathing	none	slow, irregular	normal

ankle or wrist and an injection of vitamin K is given in the thigh to prevent a serious condition called 'haemorrhagic (bleeding) disease of the newborn.' Then, if the baby has adapted well to life outside the womb, he or she is handed to the parents to hold – often for skin-to-skin contact and preliminary suckling at the mother's breast.

 ## What should a newborn look like?

When you have your first chance to see your new baby, you may notice a few variations from normal. Most newborns are, quite frankly, a bit ugly (except to Mum and Dad!). A baby born a few weeks early is often covered with fine hair called 'lanugo' (this will disappear in a week or two) and may have a thick cheesy material, the *vernix caseosa*, over much of the body (this will be removed during the first bath). If the baby has had a bit of oxygen shortage during labour, there is occasionally some sticky dark green or black material from the bowels, called 'meconium,' on the skin. You may notice some pearly white or yellow spots on the face, called 'milia (sebaceous gland hyperplasia),' which look like pimples or pustules – these will disappear in a few weeks. Some infants develop a fluctuating whole-body rash called 'erythema toxicum,' which resembles little pimples with red rims – this too will be gone in a few days without treatment. Many normal newborns have some degree of cyanosis (blue colour) in their hands and feet and around the mouth, due to their immature blood circulation. You may notice that your baby's head has a weird shape, especially if you had a long, difficult labour; this is caused by moulding during the birth process, especially at the back ('cone head'), and is called 'caput succedaneum.' You may see a fluctuating mass at one side of the head, not crossing the mid-line, caused by some bleeding under the scalp, called a 'cephalhaematoma.' The odd shape will disappear in days, and the scalp bulge in a few weeks. You may notice that your baby looks bow-legged and that his or her feet turn in; this is due to the baby's position in the womb, and will gradually correct itself by about age two.

 ## Will the baby be kept in a nursery?

Most hospitals allow healthy newborn infants to 'room in' with their mothers, as long as there are no concerns or complications that require monitoring in the neonatal intensive care unit. The nurse or midwife is trained to look after both the mother and her baby, and to teach the parents the basics of infant care – especially to help get breast-feeding established. The doctor or midwife will carry out a more complete examination of the baby before the baby goes home, answer any questions, and arrange follow-up after discharge.

How much can a newborn do?

Your new baby's nervous system has a number of unique features, many of which help an infant adapt to the outside world. These are called 'primitive reflexes.' One is the Moro or 'startle' reflex: a sudden noise or disturbance will cause the baby's arms and hands to open and move in a sort of embrace. The suckling reflex is another: if the infant's cheek is brushed, the baby turns to face that side and suckles (this is important to know when you're breast-feeding). There's the grasp reflex: when an object is placed in the baby's hand, the hand automatically closes over it; and the walking reflex: when the infant is held upright with the feet just touching a surface, one foot after the other will be placed down, simulating walking. Also, the infant is able to fix his or her eyes on special, interesting, close-up objects such as a parent's face. Except for this last one, these primitive reflexes gradually disappear by nine months of age.

What other tests are done in hospital?

Newborns in New Zealand are screened, by a heel-prick blood test, for seven diseases that, if not detected and treated in the first two or three weeks of life, can result in severe and permanent mental retardation. Without a blood test these problems are hard to find. The test is best done after your baby has been feeding for two days.

If the baby goes home before that, the test can be done at discharge and repeated two or three days later. It's most important that all babies have the screening test soon after they are born so that fast action can be taken if needed.

Only a very few babies (around 30 out of 60,000 births in New Zealand each year) will have one of these rare problems. About one in 100 babies will need a second test, this is usually because the blood wasn't taken correctly on the first test. The diseases tested for are:

1. Biotinadase Deficiency (one in 50,000 babies)
2. Congenital Adrenal Hyperplasia (one in 20,000 babies)
3. Cystic Fibrosis (one in 3,000 babies)
4. Galactosaemia (one in 120,000 babies)
5. Hypothyroidism (one in 4,500 babies)

6. Maple Syrup Urine Disease (one in 250,000 babies)

7. Phenylketonuria (one in 15,000 babies)

More information about these tests can be obtained from the New Zealand Genetic Service. Phone 09 631 0705, PO Box 872, Auckland.

 Why do some newborns look yellowish?

Jaundice – yellowing of a baby's skin and eyeballs – is very common; 60 to 70 percent of full-term newborns show some visible jaundice. In the great majority of cases it's a harmless normal variation (physiological jaundice) and needs no special treatment. Physiological jaundice appears after 24 hours of age and is more common in premature and breast-fed infants. The yellow colour comes from a pigment called 'bilirubin,' and is thought to be due to delayed maturing of the chemical processes in the liver that break down the normal end-products of red blood cells. There is controversy as to whether this type of jaundice is ever dangerous; very occasional adverse results have been reported. The most common treatment is a procedure called 'phototherapy,' in which the infant is placed in an incubator or special blanket and exposed to certain wavelengths of light that decrease the jaundice. This sometimes results in a couple of extra days in hospital or, rarely, readmission.

Sometimes, however, the accumulation of bilirubin is caused by specific disease processes (pathological jaundice) and can lead to serious consequences. The one doctors worry about most is called 'kernicterus' and involves damage to the brain resulting in hearing loss, mental retardation, and certain types of cerebral palsy, or even death. Kernicterus is now fortunately quite rare. Pathological jaundice often appears in less than 24 hours and can be the result of a large number of causes, including mother–infant blood incompatibility; bacterial infection; and various metabolic, viral, or structural diseases of the liver. The doctor must be aware of all the possibilities and begin appropriate tests in a timely fashion. Treatment may include an exchange transfusion, in which most of the infant's blood is temporarily replaced and the bilirubin is removed. Great care is now given to ensure that blood and blood products are free of infectious agents such as HIV and the hepatitis virus. Even so, doctors are very careful to do exchange transfusions only when the baby's life or brain is at risk.

The debate over circumcision

Routine male newborn circumcision (surgical removal of the foreskin) is a very controversial, often emotional subject. Some families and doctors are vehemently opposed, while others are strongly in favour. It is usually unnecessary although a few of those not circumcised at birth will need to have the procedure done later because of medical complications. In 1989 the American Academy of Pediatrics task force on neonatal circumcision adopted a policy that the procedure 'has potential medical benefits and advantages as well as disadvantages and risks.' For details on these, see Chapter 8, 'Painful Urination.'

If you decide to have your baby circumcised for medical, cultural or religious reasons remember that it is a painful procedure and that adequate anaesthesia (pain relief) should be provided.

 How long should a newborn and mother stay in hospital?

The Government has been wrestling with the spiralling cost of health care and the diminishing dollars available to pay for it. One of the strategies for reducing hospital costs is early discharge of the normal newborn; most normal full-term babies and their mothers are now discharged after 48 hours. Early discharge may interfere with the appropriate timing for screening blood tests, since some of the more common problems don't become obvious until the second or third day of life – for example, jaundice, congenital heart disease, infection, certain genetic metabolic diseases, and feeding problems. In addition, it may be difficult to teach a mother and her family how to care for and breast-feed a baby in such a short time. Careful follow-up at home by a midwife, GP or plunket nurse is very important in the first weeks of life.

 What happens when a baby is born prematurely?

Preterm birth is usually defined as less than 37 weeks' gestation, with birth weight less than 2.5 kg (5.5 pounds). Premature babies previously had significant risks of chest diseases and brain damage; in the last 20 years, however, these risks have lessened substantially. Now, with proper care, many premature babies with a gestational age as low as 28 weeks and a birth weight as low as 1 kg (2.2 pounds) grow into normal children.

If the premature baby is doing well as far as breathing and feeding are concerned, and if the birth weight is not too low (at least 1.8 kg, or four

21

pounds), the baby is usually not transferred to a special care nursery or neonatal intensive care unit. Once there is a reasonable weight gain (10 to 30 gm per day for at least three days), and the baby has no difficulty maintaining normal pink colour and normal body temperature on his or her own, the baby may be discharged. If there are breathing and/or feeding problems, or if the weight is less than 1.8 kg, referral to a special care nursery, where there are specially trained staff and technology such as respirators, may be necessary. The duration of stay in the special care nursery depends on how long it takes the baby to breathe normally and gain weight appropriately; it varies from weeks to months.

What do I do about the cord after I go home?

The umbilical cord should be kept as clean and dry as possible. It will fall off in 4 to 6 days if it dries quickly, and in 7 to 10 days if it remains a bit moist. If the skin around the cord becomes inflamed or if there is an odour or a discharge of pus, call your doctor.

The baby's first bath should always be carried out under the supervision of an experienced person. Daily bathing can be at any convenient time, except immediately after the baby's feeding.

CHAPTER 3

Working Together with Health Professionals

●●●

Once your baby is born, one of the important rituals of parenting is the well-child visit. Each appointment serves as a milestone marking your child's progress. Probably before you realise it, your little baby will have become a teenager who presents you with a new set of concerns just as challenging as those of infancy. Regularly scheduled checkups provide an excellent opportunity to review your child's growth, current development, and future needs, both physical and emotional. These visits also offer you a chance to deal with any doubts or concerns you may have.

 What happens at a well-child visit?

Each checkup is unique, as its style depend upon your child's age. Yet the goals of all these well-health visits are much the same. The doctor or nurse wants to identify and help treat any physical, developmental, or behavioural problems that may exist, so a careful medical history will be part of every checkup. The doctor or nurse may provide advice on more general topics, such as nutrition and accident prevention. Any specific concerns that remain unanswered can be addressed. Finally, immunisations are discussed and administered according to the recommended guidelines.

How often should I take my child for a well-child visit?

During infancy, your baby will experience a number of remarkable changes over just a few months. Because you need to keep abreast of these developments, and to ensure proper immunisation, you should be in contact with your baby's well-child nurse (or doctor) regularly during this period. Ideally the frequency of these visits will result in a successful relationship; the better your communication is with the health care team, the better your child's care is likely to be. As your child grows older, the intervals between well-child visits grow longer. In New Zealand each child is entitled to 12 free well-child checks; at birth, 24 hours, five days, 2 to 4 weeks, six weeks, three months, five months, nine months, 15 months, two years, three years and five years. These checks are undertaken by a well-child provider. This may be a midwife, plunket nurse, general practitioner, practice nurse or community health worker. The checks will be recorded in your baby's Well Child Tamariki Ora Health Book.

 ### When do I start these visits?

Until recently, a new mother would spend a number of days in hospital recovering from childbirth and learning how to care for her newborn; now most mothers and babies go home after just a day or two, or even a few hours. The comfort of being in your own home is undoubtedly welcome, but a number of issues must be addressed. For example, it's unlikely that breast-feeding will be established in the first 48 hours. Some parents are concerned that their infant isn't getting enough milk; others fear that the baby is too jaundiced. On a few occasions, these worries are justified. Obviously, it's better to nip any problems in the bud. Thus it is recommended that the first three checks are undertaken during the baby's first week of life, especially if the baby has been discharged from the hospital early.

At these early checks, you will be encouraged to tell your doctor, midwife or nurse how you're feeling, not only about your baby, but also about the demands of parenting. Suggestions to help with breast-feeding will be offered, if needed. The health professional will ask about the frequency of the baby's urination and, if you have a little boy, the force of the urinary stream, since a poor stream may be an early sign of obstruction. Stooling patterns will also be reviewed. Your baby will be weighed, measured, and carefully examined for any late-presenting birth defect. They will advise you of normal patterns of sleep and feeding; most newborns sleep for about three hours at a stretch and are then wakeful for about an hour, wanting to be fed. You should discuss child-safety issues related to sleep position, cot safety, and bathwater temperature.

Some well-deserved words of encouragement will generally be offered. You may also be reminded to try to pace yourself a bit. *Parenting is not a sprint – it's a marathon!*

Sudden infant death syndrome (SIDS)

S IDS, or 'cot death,' is a tragic disorder that causes the sudden, totally un-expected death of an apparently healthy infant, usually between one and four months of age. It seems that the children just stop breathing, often while asleep. Studies have suggested some contributing factors to SIDS, but we still don't under-stand exactly what goes wrong. It does not seem to be genetic.

As more is learned about the disorder, it appears some of the deaths attributed to SIDS in the past were in fact due to other causes.

Our understanding of SIDS is devel-oping rapidly. Ask your doctor for the latest information on risks for this disorder, and keep in mind that second-hand smoke appears to be a factor, as does sleeping your baby on his or her tummy. But try not to dwell on the threat; despite all the press coverage, the risk of cot death is very low.

The six-week visit: By now, your baby will display the distinctive behaviour and temperament that make him or her a unique individual. Although you may not yet feel like an expert on child care, you certainly know more about your own baby than anybody else does.

This is an important time to discuss your comfort level with parenting. If your child is having irregular feeding or sleeping patterns, if the baby is colicky, or if you feel tired and overwhelmed, share those feelings. That way, you and your doctor can manage them as a team.

Once again, your baby will be weighed and measured to make certain that growth is satisfactory, and examined for appropriate responsiveness. Any new problems such as thrush or nappy rash will be addressed (see Chapter 10, 'Skin: Spots and Rashes'). You will likely be advised that night waking is still to be expected, and that you shouldn't rush the introduction of solid foods. Finally, after a discussion of the advantages and potential side-effects, the baby will be offered immunisations against diphtheria, tetanus, pertussis, Haemophilus influenzae type B, hepatitis B and polio.

The three-month visit: By now, your baby should appear curious about the world, and eager to be part of it. The nurse or doctor will check that developmental changes are progressing on schedule. As in all well-baby checkups, a careful physical examination will be done to identify any health problems.

··
New Zealand immunisation schedule
··

Age	Disease	Vaccine
6 weeks	Diphtheria, tetanus and pertussis Hib and hepatitis B Poliomyelitis	DTPa (INFANRIX) HibPRP-OMP + Hep B (COMVAX) OPV – Sabin vaccine
3 months	Diphtheria, tetanus and pertussis Hib and hepatitis B Poliomyelitis	DTPa (INFANRIX) HibPRP-OMP + Hep B (COMVAX) OPV – Sabin vaccine
5 months	Diphtheria, tetanus and pertussis Hib and hepatitis B Poliomyelitis	DTPa (INFANRIX) Hep B (H-B-VAX II) OPV – Sabin vaccine
15 months	Diphtheria, tetanus, pertussis and Hib Measles, mumps and rubella	DTPaHibPRP-T (INFANRIX-Hib) MMR (M-M-R II)
11 years	Measles, mumps and rubella Poliomyelitis Tetanus and diphtheria (adult)	MMR (M-M-R II) OPV – Sabine vaccine Td (DiTe ANATOXAL BERNA)

● Babies who will be living in households where there are *either* recent
immigrants from high incidence countries *or* persons with current or
past history of tuberculosis should be offered BCG at birth.

Because most infants are starting to reach by this age and will soon start
to roll, safety at the change table will be highlighted. Next, it's time for
immunisations again. You will review how the last injections were tolerated,
and then the second vaccines will be offered. Before you leave, be sure to
ask any questions you may still have.

The five-month visit: By now, you're probably feeling quite comfortable
with parenting. Although time seems to have flown by, chances are you
barely remember when you weren't a parent. Most children are ready for the
introduction of solids between four and six months of age, so you will be
discussing how best to accomplish this. (See Chapter 12, 'Feeding Your
Child.') You may be thinking of returning to work outside the home, or you
may have already done so. Thus this visit may be a good time to discuss

---

Second-hand smoke and your child

Parents who smoke have usually tried stopping – even before becoming parents. There are certain risks to children exposed to second-hand smoke that parents should be aware of. The possibility of sudden infant death syndrome (SIDS, also called cot death) is greater in young infants exposed to second-hand smoke. The risk of recurrent ear infec-tions is also greater. Finally, children with asthma may have more attacks when exposed to second-hand smoke. Sometimes just knowing what their smoking may do to their children is enough for parents to get the help they need from their doctor to quit. If you can't quit, try not to smoke in your home or close to your child.

---

what to look for in daycare or a babysitter. Other issues usually addressed at this visit include teething and sleep problems. Teething seems the most variable and, arguably, the least important of infant milestones; most children get their first tooth around six months, but others appear in no rush. A few children are still waking in the night, while others who used to sleep through have reverted to getting up. The five-month checkup is a good time to review normal childhood sleep patterns and develop effective strategies for any sleep disturbance. (See Chapter 9, 'Sleeping Patterns and Problems.') After the physical examination, the third immunisations will be offered. During this visit, you may discuss safety issues such as infant walkers and the danger of small objects reaching a baby's mouth.

The nine-month visit: This visit coincides with rapid developmental change. Instead of needing the world to be brought within reach, the infant acquires the mobility to explore everything, with great curiosity. The thrust of this visit will be to evaluate how well your baby is acquiring these motor skills, and how sociable and communicative he or she has become.

Although child-safety advice is a feature of most well-baby visits, the nine-month checkup in particular tries to guarantee that mobility will lead to discovery and not tragedy. The use of stairway gates and the dangers of electrical cords will likely be discussed. Since the nine-month examination covers the introduction of finger foods, the risk of choking on certain foods may be pointed out. The visit should prompt a thorough review of household safety.

No vaccinations are required at this visit.

The 15-month visit: Once again, your baby will be measured, weighed, and examined to check that physical growth is progressing satisfactorily. By now, protection from maternal antibodies has worn off and the baby has been exposed to a variety of germs in places such as daycare. How he or she has dealt with these early-childhood illnesses will be reviewed.

Development will again be assessed. Most children are walking, using their fingers to feed themselves, handling a cup, and starting to use a few words by this time. Some are showing their assertiveness very clearly: their ability to protest loudly may have become a finely developed skill!

Immunisations against measles, mumps and rubella will be offered as well as booster shots for diphtheria, tetanus, pertussis and haemophilus type B.

The two-year visit: Developmental issues will likely dominate this checkup. By this stage the toddler is acquiring increasing verbal skills. Most have learned 50 words or more and are using short phrases such as 'What's that?' Your doctor will ask how your child is progressing in this regard, and answer any questions about diet. The use of a toothbrush, at least in imitation of other family members, may be encouraged. You will likely discuss toilet-training at this time.

It's important to realise that strong food preferences will likely have developed. Try to remember that a dislike of broccoli is not fatal. If your child seems to hate vegetables, he or she is not alone. Your doctor or nurse will likely point out that a child of this age doesn't require huge quantities of food. It's best to present a balanced diet, and to avoid too much milk or juice.

Your child's increasing autonomy will be an issue when it comes to discipline. Children at this age resist limits, however reasonable they may seem. Yet establishing consistent, reasonable limits is important for your happiness as well as your child's. Developing bedtime routines and strategies for dealing with temper tantrums will be well worth the effort. This age does not have to be the 'Terrible Twos.'

Often, at this visit, parents seek their doctor's opinion about preschool programmes. Keep in mind that the important part of a toddler's curriculum is not gymnastics, painting, or swimming, but developing the social skills to get along well with others.

The three-year visit: At this visit the nurse or doctor will assess how well your child is acquiring the developmental skills needed to function well in the world outside your home. By now, children should be talking in short sentences. For many youngsters at this stage, ideas come more rapidly than they can be expressed: stuttering is common but, fortunately, is usually temporary. Toilet-training has been achieved in about 90 percent of three-year-olds, which is a blessing. Furthermore, discipline is usually managed with less of a struggle than previously, as the concept of consequences begins to sink in. If any of these areas of development presents concerns, they should be addressed at this visit.

Sleep problems may still be an issue, but generally the cause is different. The earlier sleep disorders reflect separation anxiety, whereas now the problem may be a very vivid imagination. A three-year-old's fantasy world seems as real as the actual one. A little one may need some help dealing with the monsters and demons that tend to crop up in nightmares.

As before, height and weight will be recorded, and a physical examination carried out. Girls of this age may complain of vaginal discomfort or itching, perhaps because of inefficient early attempts at toiletting. This problem should be sensitively managed. In addition, an attempt may be made to assess both vision and blood pressure more accurately. By the end of this examination, your child may actually enjoy having a checkup.

The five year visit: This visit occurs around the time of school entry. Although it's a complete exam, the prime focus is on school readiness. How well a child sees (including colour differentiation), how well he or she listens, and how the fine motor skills have developed will all be carefully assessed. Guidelines on watching television may also be discussed.

This checkup will also focus on the child's general maturity, activity level, and temperament. You will describe how your youngster plays with other children, responds to discipline and limits, and accepts separation from parents, and whether his or her general approach to situations is a positive or negative one.

The child-safety issues mentioned will reflect this stage of increased independence. Does your child know your address and telephone number? Is he or she prepared to respond to strangers appropriately?

 Once my child is in school, do these exams continue?

School age children are usually seen when health concerns arise. You may wish to arrange a regular well-child check with your doctor or nurse. Your nurse or doctor will see himself or herself as an advocate for your youngster, so don't hesitate to share any concerns about education, behaviour, or attention span.

A physical examination may be performed. At this stage, most children – male or female – tend to be quite shy about being examined. This is natural, and your nurse or doctor will respond sensitively.

Athletics tend to become more and more important at this age. You may discuss community sports programmes and enrolling your child in swim classes; you will likely talk about bicycle safety and in-line skating. Far too many children die needlessly, or suffer serious injury, because basic safety precautions have been overlooked or rejected.

Checkups may continue into the preadolescent years. The well-child visits help firm the bonds between the doctor, nurse and the child. Children at this age are usually terrific – enthusiastic about their team sports and all extracurricular activities. Energy and creativity abound, and their *joie de vivre* is infectious.

Sometimes, however, this stage is not the bed of roses it should be. Difficulties at school, troubles with peers, and coping with parental separation or remarriage can cloud a child's emotions. If a youngster appears to be struggling with a problem, this visit may serve as a catalyst to seeking a solution. Vision and hearing is tested routinely in schools, in New Zealand. You should receive a report of the results of these tests after they are done.

Physical examinations include the continued monitoring of height and weight. Vision is checked again, as nearsightedness may appear at this age. Any early signs of puberty will be noted and reassurance provided, particularly to young boys who notice firm little lumps under their nipples (this is simply breast tissue, which will disappear over time). The spine will be checked for abnormal curvature, which appears first in preadolescence.

At 11 years children should receive booster immunisations against tetanus-diphtheria, measles-mumps-rubella (MMR) and polio.

What about the teen years?

Adolescence presents a challenge for both parents and doctors. Sometimes it helps to remember that this period is turbulent for the adolescent as well. It's a time of great change, both physically and behaviourally. When we are children, for better or worse, our value system depends largely upon that of our parents. Adults, on the other hand, should have a clear idea of who they are and what is really important to them. The transformation from child to adult, during which unwanted values are discarded and replaced by the young person's own adult choices, constitutes the great developmental task of adolescence. The whole process necessarily involves experimentation and rebellion. Most teens, if they are honest with themselves, find the period difficult and unsettling.

Well-health visits during adolescence should be framed by these realities. A frank discussion about confidentiality and privacy is usually a good idea, and both the parents and the adolescent should be involved. Patient care tends to be best when good communication exists between the doctor and the patient. This can be more easily accomplished when the teenage patient trusts that any discussion will be confidential. With this privilege comes some degree of responsibility: it should be the adolescent's job to attend appointments on time. Like most dealings with teenagers, the visits will be less stressful if the rules and policies are discussed in advance and found to be mutually agreeable.

Much of the physical examination of teens during their health-maintenance visits tends to deal with issues of puberty. For females, this involves monitoring the onset of menstruation and possibly managing irregular or painful periods. A clear and open-ended invitation to discuss contraception should be issued to the teenager. Most nurses and doctors try to handle the issues related to adolescent sexuality in a non-threatening and supportive fashion.

In early adolescence, a number of children, especially boys, lag behind their peers in both growth and sexual maturation. This can be quite troubling; it's hard on a child to look 10 years old when some classmates can pass for 17. It's also a challenge to compete athletically with such a size disadvantage. Fortunately, time is a great equaliser, and catch-up growth is the rule.

Some diseases – inflammatory bowel disease, for example – begin very gradually, and poor weight gain can be the first sign. A weight check will also provide an opportunity to discuss another problem of adolescence: eating disorders. How teens perceive their size and shape, and what they eat, are important topics that should be addressed during these visits.

A number of other physical issues are particularly important to the adolescent. What teens see in the mirror is not what the rest of us notice. Acne is perceived as a curse more dreadful than the great plagues, and working out an effective but not excessive treatment plan is one of the goals at teen examinations. These visits also serve the adolescent athlete, who is sometimes required to undergo a physical exam before participating in a team sport.

What about the adolescent with a chronic illness or disability? Most teens with an ongoing problem simply wish their disease would disappear so they could be like everyone else. One response they sometimes fall into is ignoring some or even all of their treatment. It's crucial for the doctor to let the teenager vent his or her feelings about living with asthma, diabetes, epilepsy, or whatever the chronic problem happens to be. If possible, the patient with a chronic illness must be persuaded that complying with the treatment plan is the best way to ensure as normal a life as possible.

More teenage girls are taking up smoking than ever before, perhaps because they think that it's 'cool' or that it will help them control their weight. Nagging doesn't work, but information about the known risks may. A doctor can explain how smoking reduces cardiovascular fitness. It may also help – especially with girls – to remind them of the strong odour of smoking, and the smelly residue left on hair and clothes.

Many teens don't realise that smoking is more than just a cancer risk; it's also a major risk for heart disease, and lung diseases such as emphysema. The most important factor in cutting down heart disease in the last 30 years has been the fact that many fewer males are smoking than before; it is tragic that this saving of lives is offset by the increase in female smoking.

As with nutrition and exercise, the best argument you can offer is your own example. It's difficult to make a convincing case against smoking with a pack of cigarettes in your pocket!

Again, some advice on safety is in order. Accidental injury, and even death, remain the greatest danger to the well-being of most teenagers. Even if the impact is slight, most doctors feel that providing some advice on safety is a key part of an adolescent's annual exam. (Chapter 13 provides a thorough summary of safety precautions for various ages.) In the later teen years, a candid conversation about alcohol use, particularly in the context of social events, is worthwhile. Even getting a teen to pledge not to ride home with a driver who has been drinking is an important step in promoting responsible behaviour. For doctors as well as parents, it's best to remember that with teenagers, discussions work much better than lectures.

Q What about side-effects of all these immunisations?

It's hard to imagine a world in which thousands of helpless children suffocated in their own bodily secretions because they had contracted diphtheria, or lay paralysed in an iron-lung machine because of polio, or died of measles-related pneumonia. Yet that is how things were. The development of immunisations has dramatically reduced the occurrence of such preventable tragedies. It remains one of humankind's great achievements.

Still, these miracle preventives can have side-effects – some minor, some serious – as indicated below. For information on the diseases themselves, see Chapter 14, 'Diseases and Medical Conditions.'

Chickenpox The vaccine is licensed for use in New Zealand, available for those who wish to purchase it, but not free on the national schedule. It is live, attenuated (specially grown and weakened) vaccine. The vaccine is well tolerated, with very few significant side-effects. Five percent of children get a fever 10 to 14 days after inoculation, but only a few of these develop a rash. In teens, a rash is slightly more common.

The **diphtheria** vaccine, diphtheria toxoid, is a preparation of diphtheria toxin inactivated by formaldehyde. Infants generally tolerate the inoculation well, but temporary local reactions (soreness and redness) and fever may occur. These side-effects are more common in older children, so the vaccine for this age group is adjusted to contain less toxoid.

Hepatitis B immunisation uses a vaccine made from genetically engineered purified hepatitis B protein. The vaccine cannot cause hepatitis. No serious complications from the vaccine have been reported in children, but local irritation at the site of the injection, low-grade fever, and irritability occur in approximately 10 percent of cases.

The **Haemophilus (Hib)** vaccine is remarkably safe. Fever and local irritation occur at rates similar to those following injection with a harmless placebo, and no severe life-threatening reactions have been associated with the vaccine.

The vaccines developed to combat **measles, mumps,** and **rubella** are routinely given as a combined MMR injection. They are live, attenuated vaccines, intended to create an infection so mild that no clinical symptoms result and yet lifelong immunity is induced. This protection is obtained in the great majority of children.

Fever and a temporary rash occur in about 10 percent of vaccine recipients, usually around 10 days after the inoculation. Sore joints, thought to be due to the rubella component, are occasionally noted after a few weeks, but this is much more likely in older patients, especially women. Other side-effects, ranging from tingling fingers to encephalitis, are extremely rare.

The live MMR vaccines must be given with caution to, or even withheld from, children with immune deficiencies or a sensitivity to certain elements of the vaccines such as neomycin. Allergy to eggs is no longer a contraindication to MMR vaccine but caution is required. Administration of MMR should be delayed if the child has a severe acute illness, but not for minor acute illness, even if fever is present.

The **pertussis** (whooping cough) vaccine is prepared from purified components of the organism and is called acellular pertussis vaccine. There is the risk of side-effects; however, the incidence of these is much lower than the previously used whole cell pertussis vaccine. Minor local reactions at the site of the injection, or fever and fussiness, occur in up to 30 percent of the recipients. Fortunately, these problems disappear on their own in a day or two. Rarely, persistent and inconsolable crying that lasts for hours follows pertussis vaccination. Convulsions or a state of limp unresponsiveness have been reported in approximately one out of 1,750 recipients of the old (whole cell) vaccine. Most of these convulsions are brief and related to fever; neither these nor seizures unaccompanied by fever have been implicated in producing later epilepsy.

In the past there has been widespread fear about a possible association of severe neurological disease and the pertussis vaccine. The problem has been exhaustively studied and debated. Permanent neurological damage does *not* appear to be caused by the vaccine and, if it were, the increased occurrence would be so slight as to be essentially unmeasurable. Note that brain damage, and even death, can result from getting the actual disease.

Any child who has had a severe allergic reaction to the pertussis vaccine should not have another dose. If an episode of reduced responsiveness or marked listlessness occurred shortly after the vaccination, the relative risks of further immunisation must be considered, and you should discuss further with your doctor or nurse.

Some conditions that were once felt to be reasons to avoid DTP immunisation are no longer considered enough of a risk to interfere with complete vaccination. These include high fever within 48 hours of inoculation, persistent crying, or a prior history of seizures that are now controlled. Also, a minor viral illness such as the common cold, even if accompanied by fever, need not delay the vaccination.

If you give your child paracetamol around the time of injection, side-effects such as fever, irritability, and local reaction may be significantly diminished. A new type of pertussis vaccine (acellular vaccine) is now used and may provide protection with fewer reactions. For now, one thing is clear: children are at greater risk when they remain unimmunised than when they are properly vaccinated.

Two different methods of **polio** protection are available, inactivated (IPV) and live oral (OPV) polio virus vaccine. Both are effective in preventing the disease caused by the three different strains of polio virus. The vaccine currently in use is the OPV. OPV contains live virus and can cause vaccine-associated paralysis on very rare occasions; the risk to vaccine recipients is estimated at one case per 11.7 million doses of distributed vaccine, and the risk to people in contact with those vaccinated is calculated at about one case per three million doses. OPV should never be administered to immunodeficient children, those on medication that interferes with immunity, or children closely associated with such vulnerable individuals. All immunosuppressed people and their contacts should be offered injectable polio vaccine (IVP). The side-effects of the current IPV shots are minimal and essentially limited to minor local reactions. Immunising children whose mothers are pregnant, however, presents no risk to the unborn children.

Immunisation against **tetanus** is with tetanus toxoid, which is tetanus toxin treated with formaldehyde and combined with an aluminum salt. Adverse reactions to primary immunisation are quite rare.

CHAPTER 4

Crying: How Much Is Normal?

 Have you been in the annoying situation of having a car alarm sound and sound? What about one of those house alarms that seems to go on and on? The sound is meant to be unpleasant, but it's also supposed to alert us to the fact that there's a problem. Yet sometimes the sound continues and nobody seems to be dealing with the cause. This is rather like taking care of a baby who continually cries and fusses and seems to be telling us that something's the matter, when we can't 'turn off the alarm.' We're frustrated at not being able to establish what all the noise means, let alone solve the problem. It distresses us that we can't help the baby. After all, isn't that what a parent is supposed to do?

Of course, all babies cry and fuss from time to time. Unfortunately, some of them do so a lot more than others – especially in the first few months of life.

How much do most babies cry? At what age do they cry most?

In a study done by the well-known American paediatrician Dr. T. Berry Brazelton, 80 mothers were asked to keep daily records of their infants' crying for the first 12 weeks of life. In each 24-hour period, they indicated what the baby was doing at various times (crying, feeding, sleeping, sucking, being held). Whenever the baby cried, they noted the type of cry (sudden or gradual), what relieved it and for how long, and what seemed to have caused it.

Dr. Brazelton chose mothers who seemed to have a normal, positive approach to mothering; more than half had more than one child, were known to him personally, and were described as relaxed and competent.

The study showed that crying increased from an hour and 45 minutes per day at two weeks of age to a peak of two hours and 45 minutes at six weeks, and then gradually diminished to less than an hour by 12 weeks.

What time of day do babies cry most?

Dr. Brazelton found that in three-week-old infants, the fussing was spread through the day but there was a strong tendency to cry between 6:00 and 11:00 P.M. By six weeks there was occasional crying in the early morning, but most fussing occurred later in the day; some babies began around noon, many cried between 6:00 and 8:00 P.M., and a few were crying after 2:00 A.M. By 10 weeks of age the babies had quieted down considerably; what little crying they did was mostly between 6:00 A.M. and noon, or between 4:30 and 10:30 in the evening.

What's the difference between 'fussing' and crying?

When babies cry because they are hungry or wet, you can generally soothe them by solving the problem – with a feeding, a dry nappy, or whatever. The term 'fussing' is generally applied to crying that goes on for no apparent reason; the child rejects a pacifier or dummy and other proffered solutions, and may quiet briefly if picked up or rocked, but starts crying again when this attention is removed. Fussing is frustrating for parents because they feel that the child must want something, yet they can't figure out what it is.

If that's fussing, then what is 'colic'?

'Colic' – sometimes called 'three-month colic' – is indicated by a more extreme degree of fussing. It has been described as 'bursts of irritability, fussing, or crying lasting for a total of more than three hours a day and occurring on more than three days in any one week, for at least three weeks.' But colic also seems to involve a far more intense and angry type of fussing, which is acutely distressing to parents. Mothers can be so upset by the persistent crying of a colicky baby that they begin to lose their milk; the persistent frustration and helplessness can create serious tensions in the rest of the family, which may in turn increase the baby's fussing.

Since colic seems to be an extension of fussing, it may be simpler to think of it as 'heavy fussing.' It's important to keep in mind that in almost all cases, no physical cause for the crying can be found; moreover, there is no reason to believe that the amount of crying puts the child at risk of any complication, or that somehow reducing the crying would help the baby in any physical way.

Frequently, fussy babies (particularly heavy fussers) don't just cry a lot; they have all kinds of extreme responses that make them generally more difficult to deal with. It seems that infants who cry excessively are also more sensitive, more irritable, and less easily soothed than average, and that they are more than usually active. Dr. Brazelton found further differences: for example, the lighter fussers tended to spend a lot more time sucking their fingers and pacifiers, whereas pacifiers or dummies didn't seem to placate the heavy fussers.

 Could these heavy fussers be reacting to tension in their homes?
From his study of colicky babies with relaxed, experienced mothers, Dr. Brazelton concluded that heavy fussing did not necessarily indicate any neglect or abnormality in parenting.

It's more likely the other way around: the baby's constant fussing can put heavy stress on the parents, who then fall into reproaching themselves (or worse, each other) about their parenting abilities. Sometimes they refuse to give themselves a break and leave the baby with someone else. This guilty response is understandable but irrational, and it can only make matters worse; parents who find themselves slipping into it should discuss the problem with their general practitioner or midwife.

 Is it possible that the baby would fuss less if I responded differently?
In one three-group study, parents were given different instructions. The first group, the parents of 200 newborns, were given no special instructions. The second group, the parents of 70 newborns, were given the following instructions:

1. Try never to let your baby cry.

2. In working out the reason for his crying consider the following possibilities:

    a) The baby is hungry and wants to be fed.

    b) The baby is not hungry but wants to suck.

    c) The baby wants to be held and cuddled.

    d) The baby is bored and wants some stimulation – singing, smiling, talking, or play.

    e) The baby is tired and wants to sleep.

3. If the crying continues for more than five minutes of using one approach, then try another.

4. Work out your own way of exploring all the possibilities above.

 38

The third group, the parents of another 70 newborns, were given baby slings and asked to carry their babies three more hours each day. All of these infants were monitored, using diaries, audio recordings, and questionnaires, and all the parents followed instructions, but no significant difference was found; regardless of the intervention, the infants fussed just as much.

In another study, it was found that if non-colicky babies were carried more, there was a 43 percent reduction in crying and fussing; however, it seems that colicky babies continue to cry, regardless of how much they are carried.

Since fussy babies often seem to be consoled by car motion, some parents assume that repetitive movements, vibrations, and 'white noise' may do the same. But a study tested this by comparing three groups of fussy babies; parents in one group were given a device that vibrates the crib and makes a soft background noise, and those in another group were told to respond in the same way as the second group in the three-group study. The amount of fussing and the degree of parental stress improved with time, regardless of which group the families were in.

In short, no matter how much we try to soften the fussier babies' interaction with the environment, they cry just as much.

Colic: Looking for a Cause

Many factors have been suggested as reasons for colic – some external, such as parental stress, and some internal, such as digestive problems. But so far no theory has been convincingly supported by scientific studies.

 Could the colic be due to an allergy to cow's milk or soya milk?
An allergic reaction to cow's milk is a specific medical condition in which the baby's body reacts very adversely to even a small amount of the protein in cow's-milk formula, or to some of the cow's-milk protein that comes through from the mother's diet in her breast milk. It's also possible to be allergic to the soya protein in soya-milk formulas. People often confuse this specific allergy with *intolerance* for the sugar in milk, which is called 'lactose' – a very different situation (see below). If the baby did have an allergy, there would be certain signs: he or she might be extremely colicky, and the colic would likely continue beyond the typical three-month mark. The baby might have diarrhoea and vomiting and might not be gaining weight well. When the stool was tested, there might be traces of blood detected, even if they weren't visible to the naked eye.

A pediatric gastroenterologist who reviewed all the studies on this subject concluded that certain studies implicating cow's-milk protein as a cause of colic were looking at that very small percentage of extremely fussy infants who had symptoms of a true allergy to cow's-milk protein. There is no reason to assume that cow's milk also bothers non-allergic babies. Indeed, there is evidence that colic is *not* usually due to an allergy. Colic also occurs equally in formula-fed and breast-fed babies.

 There seems to be so much gas in my baby's tummy. Could this be causing pain?

It's possible that all the crying and fussing result in the baby's swallowing a lot of extra air, and that this causes the gurgly tummy sounds and the excessive flatus (farting).

A number of studies have considered the possibility that colicky babies have lactose intolerance and are not completely digesting the lactose (sugar) present in breast milk or cow's milk. If this sugar is not completely digested, it passes into the lower part of the bowel; bacteria can feed on it there and produce gas. (For more information on lactose intolerance, see Chapter 12, 'Feeding Your Child.')

A soya formula does not contain lactose, and there are cow's-milk formulas in which the lactose has been altered to be more digestible. Unfortunately, some studies show that when fussy babies are fed lactose-free milk, or an artificial lactase enzyme to help them digest lactose, they still cry and fuss just as much. It seems there is no scientific basis for using these formulas in an attempt to reduce the amount of gas.

 Could my baby be fussing because food isn't moving well in the intestine and the baby is getting cramps?

There is some evidence that babies who show high levels of motilin – the substance that controls the movement in the small intestine – may go on to develop symptoms of colic. But we do not yet have conclusive evidence of a connection, and in any case there is no proven treatment for the condition, even if it is related to colic.

 Could my baby's spilling be causing discomfort that looks like colic?

If the baby vomits, turns away from the breast or bottle, screams after the feeding starts, or wakes from sleep a few hours after feeding with heavy crying, and if these symptoms become worse when one would normally expect fussiness to subside (after age three months), consider the possibility that the baby is having bad heartburn. A trial of antacids may be used in treating these babies. An Australian study has shown that most fussy babies do not have gastro-oesophageal reflux.

 ### If there's no physical problem, why does my baby cry so much?

The inconsolability is most likely part of the normal development of an infant who just a few months ago was in a completely different environment, not dependent on oral feeding or subject to changes in temperature, light, touch, etc. These infants are demonstrating their frustration with life outside the womb in the only way they can. Some infants seem to adjust very easily, whereas others struggle longer and harder. No parents, not even those with excellent responsiveness to their baby's needs, can recreate the coddled existence these babies may still recall.

Of course, we can't prove that this is the answer – yet it seems to be the only way to explain why these babies seem frustrated and angry as opposed to in pain; why studies searching for external causes produce inconclusive results (and studies on the issue of colic have filled pediatric literature for a long time); and why parents have such a difficult time settling these babies, even if they follow all the recommendations religiously.

Taking Care of a Fussy Baby

Desperate parents have tried any number of remedies to soothe their fussing babies. So far, no approach has been shown to be both safe and generally effective.

 ### Might my baby fuss less if I stopped breast-feeding?

Formula-fed infants cry just as much as breast-fed ones, so there's no reason to switch to formula. Mothers often feel that they aren't producing enough milk, or that there must be something wrong with it, but this is not usually the case. Fussy babies are just harder to feed, by breast or formula; eventually they all get sufficient milk.

When 374 healthy infants were studied from birth to six weeks, it was found that infants who were switched from breast to formula did the same amount of fussing over a 24-hour period as those who were consistently breast-fed. However, there was less evening crying in the formula-fed babies;

crying tended to be spread through the day.

If your baby has a slow, rhythmical suckle, is having at least one substantial bowel movement each day from three weeks of age, and has at least six soaked nappies a day after the fifth day, the intake of milk is likely adequate. Good weight gain is a sure sign that the baby is getting sufficient milk.

Certain foods in the mother's diet are felt by some to affect the baby – these include apricots, beans, broccoli, cabbage, onions, peaches, prunes, rhubarb, and turnips. Although these foods don't cause fussing or crying, the general recommendation is that the suspected food be withdrawn from the diet for a week just to see if that makes any difference; if not, the food should be reintroduced. Remember that a nursing mother should have a healthy, well-balanced diet, and that excluding important foods may be harmful. (For more on breast-feeding and formulas, see Chapter 12, 'Feeding Your Child.')

 ### Would it help to change the formula?

Changing the formula generally makes no scientific sense. Parents often switch the type, brand, or preparation of their baby's formula for no logical reason. If any change is noted, it probably would have happened anyway.

Switching to a hydrolysed casein/whey formula (see Chapter 13) occasionally works. Babies who have heavy fussing that goes on for more than three months, a strong family history of allergic conditions like asthma or eczema, and symptoms like diarrhoea, mucusy stools, vomiting, and/or microscopic amounts of blood in the stool (detected by a test done in your doctor's surgery) may have an allergy (mentioned above) to cow's-milk or soya protein. In these formulas the components have been broken down into smaller pieces that are less likely to cause allergic reactions. A hydrolysed casein/whey formula, which is generally a lot more expensive, should be used only on a trial basis. If it seems to work, that doesn't mean the baby is permanently allergic; the change may have been purely coincidental. Even true allergic reactions sometimes seem to disappear in a short time, so dairy and soya products should be reintroduced at a later date. It's important not to label your child 'allergic' without cause.

Another experiment parents often try is introducing other foods, like cereal, on the grounds that the baby may be hungry. Formula actually contains more calories than cereal; moreover, cereal is often difficult to introduce into a baby's mouth at this age because he or she has not yet learned to accept a spoon. Studies have shown that infants introduced to cereals don't cry any less, although they seem to feed less often.

What about all the advice people give me? Should I just ignore it?
Family, friends, and even professionals often assume that if a baby cries inconsolably, the parents must be doing something wrong. Their advice is copious, and frequently contradictory. The fact is that even first-time parents intuitively learn the best way to handle their baby, and endless input from other people is less than helpful. You may sometimes learn a useful specific tip from a book or a conversation, but don't feel obliged to try every new idea. There's a healthy balance between taking advice and having confidence in your own ability.

Remember that just because the baby is still fussing doesn't mean you've failed to provide everything. If all the baby's obvious needs have been met, it's not inappropriate to leave the child to cry. On the other hand, if you prefer to try to comfort the baby, that's fine too. Don't worry about spoiling the child at this point; you can work on establishing routines later, when you are past this stressful stage.

 Are there medicines or other remedies to treat fussing?
Medicines have been tested as treatments for colicky behaviour. They fall into two categories: either they work but aren't safe, or they don't work but parents want to believe they do.

A good example of the latter is simethicone, which is supposed to work by making it easier for the baby to release swallowed gas. A recent study shows that a placebo (a look-alike syrup) works just as well. The same holds true for gripe water; a placebo was just as 'effective.' (Note that some formulations of gripe water contain alcohol.)

There are other medicines that make the baby sleepy. Examples include alcohol, diphenhydramine hydrochloride (Benadryl), chloral hydrate, and phenobarbital. Regardless of whether these medicines work or not, it is not acceptable for a parent to decide to use them on a baby.

In a study involving 97 infants, the various ingredients of a prescribed colic mixture were tested individually against a placebo. The sedative ingredient, phenobarbital, worked no better than the placebo. Neither did the muscle relaxant, homatropine methylbromide – an atropine-like drug that relaxes the muscle in the bowel wall, and may also affect the baby's central nervous system. Neither did alcohol, which can cause convulsions in infants by making their level of blood sugar drop. Not only are these mixtures ineffective, but there have been reports of side-effects that were *acute life-threatening events* (ALTEs).

The one medicine that does improve fussy behaviour – dicyclomine hydrochloride – has also been associated with ALTEs, and is no longer used for this purpose.

Some parents are under the impression that herbal teas are safe, 'natural' remedies for colic. In fact they may contain substances that work just like the atropine-related drug described above. Although one commercially prepared tea has been studied and may be effective, that doesn't mean that others are safe; poisonings with herbal teas are frequently reported.

In short, medication – pharmaceutical or herbal – is not a safe treatment for a fussing infant.

 ### What if a colicky baby gets a real physical problem? How would I know?

Tell your doctor if you see signs of a milk or soya allergy, mentioned above, or if the baby has a fever.

If the baby is having hard and infrequent bowel movements, this suggests constipation (or holding back on bowel movements); your doctor can suggest ways to remedy that. If there are no bowel movements and the baby has any vomiting of a bright yellow or green colour, this indicates a bowel blockage, a rare occurrence that requires immediate attention.

If you detect any specific part of the baby's body that seems tender, call your doctor immediately. Examples include pain when the nappy is changed; pain with hip movement, which could be a sign of infection of the hip joint; swelling and apparent tenderness in the groin, which could indicate a twist of the testis or a twisted hernia; or tenderness along any of the arms and legs or collar-bones, which might mean a broken bone.

Of course, it's impossible for you as a parent to know whether you are under- or overreacting. The best thing to do if you're in doubt is to have your doctor examine the baby and allay your concerns once and for all. Doctors are used to parents bringing their fussy babies back to the surgery week after week. They understand that a fussy baby can be very anxiety-provoking, and that knowing nothing is really wrong can provide a great deal of reassurance.

 ### What can I do when I'm at my wits' end?

Being with a fussy baby day and night, losing more and more sleep, can make anyone exhausted and exasperated. It's essential to rely on family members and friends to give you a break. Some parents have difficulty leaving their baby, but resting (and that means being away and out of earshot) enables you to return refreshed and better able to take good care of your baby.

Above all, recognise that at times this combination of weariness and desperation may result in a dangerous situation for both parent and child. It's important to express your feelings of frustration clearly to family members, friends, and your doctor. Failing to do so can only make things worse for you. If you feel that you (or anyone else) might possibly lose control out of exasperation, *get help*. Never feel isolated; remember that there is always someone who can assist you. Parents who have recently moved to a new community can always call a plunket nurse or general practitioner.

The Long-Term Outlook

Parents often want to know if fussy babies are likely to have more difficult personalities and behaviour when they grow up. Is a calmer baby likely to grow up to be more easygoing? The short answer seems to be that fussy behaviour until about the age of three months (which is when most colicky babies settle down) is not associated with any long-term behaviour problems. Calmer babies are just as likely to be challenging at a later stage as their fussier counterparts.

What if your infant is still inconsolable beyond the four-month mark? Studies show that these infants may go on to be more challenging children, but this is not a hard-and-fast rule.

Infants who remained very fussy beyond four months of age are often described by their parents as being very active children who just won't keep still. They are very alert and often don't seem happy in one position. Parents often pick them up and put them down repetitively in an attempt to make them more comfortable. Routines are often a problem; these babies tend to fight sleep, and as they get older they may be very resistant to eating. Also, they are more likely to develop constipation because they seem to resist having a bowel movement; in other words, they hold on too long. Stubbornness seems to be a hallmark of these children, and temper tantrums are more likely.

Whereas these infants initially appeared dissatisfied, later they seem to develop a pattern of provoking the hapless parent into situations of having to say no – at which point the child acts as if the parent is mean, and seems oblivious of the course of events that obviously led to this refusal. The child may pout and generally behave like a poor, mistreated, misunderstood little thing.

Families have to follow routines: bedtime means going to sleep at a specified time, certain items can't be touched because they are fragile or dangerous, siblings have to share. All of these realities may be misused by such children to force their parents to keep saying no. They seem unmoved by reasoning, and behavioural techniques are of limited value. The parents can only deal with the issue in a practical way, and realise that a stage has been reached where the environment can no longer bend to the whim of the child. Alas, we must wait and hope that the child eventually accepts this reality. There is only so much these parents can be expected to achieve, given the limited influences at their disposal. A reasonable and consistent approach and a healthy realisation that this problem is not their fault is the best course we can suggest.

CHAPTER 5

Fever: When Is It Serious?

● ●

Fever is one of the most common reasons for parents to take their child to see a doctor; it may account for a quarter of all doctor visits for children under two years of age. Unfortunately, although there have been many significant advances in our knowledge of fever, there are many things we still don't understand. Parents' fears about fever – sometimes referred to as 'fever phobia,' and perhaps made worse by the concern shown by many doctors – may lead to unnecessary phone calls and doctor visits, improper use of fever medications, and inappropriate attempts to bring down the child's temperature at all costs. Yet while parents worry so much about fever, many children are not particularly bothered by it.

Q What is fever, and what does it mean?

The first thing to remember is that fever is a symptom, not a disease. It helps us know that something unusual is going on in the child, and it may be the first sign that the child is unwell. It's the body's normal response to bacterial and viral infections and is a very common symptom in childhood illnesses.

Normally the temperature of the body ranges between 36°C and 37.8°C (96.8°F and 100°F). A fever is defined as a temperature above the normal range, which varies slightly, depending on where on the body it's measured. A temperature is considered a fever if it's above 37.2°C (99°F) under the arm, above 37.5°C (99.5°F) in the mouth, or above 38°C (100.4°F) measured rectally. The easiest place to take your child's temperature is under the arm; although it's not the most accurate measurement, that's probably not as important as simply knowing that the child does have a fever. For practical and safety reasons, children's temperatures should not be taken orally (in the mouth) until they are over five years of age. Rectal temperatures are probably the most accurate, but the procedure may be frightening and uncomfortable for small children, and is often avoided these days. Tympanic thermometers measure core body temperatures via the ear and this is equivalent to rectal temperature. They are unreliable under 12 months of age.

 ### Is fever in children helpful, harmful, or dangerous?

There is good information from laboratory studies supporting the view that fever is actually helpful, though some doctors still believe otherwise. The body protects itself against infections caused by germs, either bacteria or viruses, by a defence system known as the 'immune response.' This defence system is thought to be helped or 'kick-started' by fever. Furthermore, the types of fever usually seen in children are not harmful; they do *not* cause brain damage or death. Although fever may cause convulsions (seizures) in some children (fewer than five percent), these convulsions are not harmful and have no long-term effects. Rare complications in children with fever are usually due to the underlying disease, such as meningitis, rather than the fever itself. Therefore, in trying to determine the seriousness of a fever, you should pay less attention to the height of the fever than to the child's behaviour. Does he or she look sick and act sick? If not, the fever probably isn't serious.

Is your child sick?

In deciding whether your child is really sick, look for these features:

Well	Sick
● lively and alert	● droopy and apathetic
● eating well	● eating poorly
● playing normally	● ignoring toys
● interested in surroundings	● uninterested in surroundings
● smiling at you	● unresponsive
● able to be comforted	● inconsolable
● normal pink colour	● pale/ashen complexion
● moist mucous membranes (inside mouth, eyelids)	● dry lips, no tears

---

Common Causes of Childhood Fever

The causes of fever vary, depending on the age of the child, and so does the seriousness of the fever.

What if my newborn baby has a fever?

In a child less than a month old, fever is often due to infection, sometimes bacterial and potentially serious. Dehydration (often the result of insufficient milk), overdressing, or an overheated environment may also cause a mild fever.

Any fever in this period requires immediate medical attention, not because of the fever itself, which is not dangerous, but because the underlying cause may be serious. Fever is often the only sign of infection in a newborn, who gives fewer warning signals of being unwell than does an older child. Other symptoms that may indicate serious illness in a newborn include a lower than normal temperature, not feeding properly, and vomiting feeds. It's particularly difficult to distinguish trivial problems from more serious illness at this age. Because of the dangers of bacterial infection, many doctors hospitalise infants less than a month old with fever, in order to observe them closely and start treatment with antibiotics while awaiting the results of lab tests. Treatment depends on how ill the baby looks, the results of blood tests, and other factors. If the lab tests are normal and the infant quickly returns to normal feeding, activity, and sleeping patterns, the hospital stay is likely to be no longer than 48 hours.

What if my baby is between one and three months old?

In this case the fever is still worrisome, but much less so. Medical views about managing fever at this age are changing; your baby may be handled at home with very close observation and follow-up, or may be admitted to hospital, depending on the circumstances. Fever at this age is usually related to viral illness, but you should seek prompt medical attention if the infant is not lively, or is not behaving normally.

What about a baby over three months but under two years?

Fever in this age group is primarily the result of viral infections in the upper respiratory tract – in other words, the common cold. The infant characteristically has a runny nose with a clear discharge, stuffiness, and a cough or congestion; he or she may vomit or have the occasional loose bowel movement. The most common complication of a viral cold is an ear infection; you

49

can often recognise this by the sudden development of irritability, crying, pulling of the ear, vomiting, or not feeding well. (Teething around six months of age may produce many of these symptoms, but it's not associated with fever.) Often the clear discharge from the nose will become thicker and turn yellow or green, which may be a sign of a secondary bacterial infection.

A very high fever (as high as 40.5°C, or 105°F) that is not accompanied by other signs of sickness, except perhaps irritability, may indicate roseola, a common viral infection at this age (see Chapter 14, 'Diseases and Medical Conditions'). Infants may also develop fever following immunisation shots.

 What about older children?

In children aged 2 to 6, viral infections remain the most common cause of fever. Other possible causes at this age include strep throat, ear infections, bronchitis, and digestive- and urinary-tract infections.

In school-age children, viral respiratory-tract infections are the most common cause of fever. Strep throat and scarlet fever (strep throat with a rash) typically occur at this age. Urinary-tract infections, particularly in girls, may cause a fever as well. Bronchitis, pneumonia, and meningitis are uncommon causes of fever in school-age children.

When to get help

Any fever at all in a newborn infant should immediately be reported to a doctor, or the baby should be taken to the nearest emergency department. Seek medical attention immediately for any child with a fever above 40.5°C (105°F) if the child is crying inconsolably, hard to awaken, or confused, or acts or looks very sick or has trouble breathing. Immediate medical aid should also be sought if the child has a stiff neck, has convulsions for the first time, or has purple spots (petechiae) anywhere on the skin. Children who have diseases such as leukemia, or who are on immunosuppressants, should also have medical help immediately if they have any fever.

In children aged three months to two years, a fever above 38.5°C (101°F) for 24 hours merits a call to the doctor during regular office hours. A fever that continues for more than three days, irrespective of the age of the child, also demands a call to the doctor's office. Other reasons to seek medical help include a fever in association with behavioural changes such as crankiness or unusual quietness, or an appearance that makes you anxious.

Treating a Fever

The most important reason for treating a child who has a fever is to make the child more comfortable. In other words, the *child* should be treated, not the thermometer. A feverish child who is not uncomfortable requires no treatment, since the fever itself isn't dangerous.

Since most fevers are viral in origin, no treatment is available for the cause. However, if the fever has a bacterial cause such as an ear infection, your doctor can determine the appropriate medication to treat the infection.

What else can I do to make my child feel better?

All children with fever should be given extra fluids to prevent dehydration from sweating. They should be dressed in less clothing than usual, and where possible their activities should be reduced. If the child feels cold and is shivering with chills, which means the temperature is rising, a light blanket may give some immediate relief. Children should *not* be bundled up to 'sweat out' the fever; this may be harmful as the body's excess heat can't escape. The room must not be overheated but rather kept at a comfortable 20° C (68° F). Children should not be covered with wet towels or sheets, which may make them uncomfortable, and alcohol sponging must never be used because the alcohol can be absorbed through the skin.

The use of lukewarm sponge baths is controversial; some studies indicate that these baths are no more effective than medication to lower the child's temperature, and in fact may make them uncomfortable with shivering and chills. (The use of sponge bathing has been abandoned in many busy emergency departments.) Other doctors feel that a tepid bath does no harm and may be a useful technique for parents who are anxious to 'do something.' If you do decide to try a sponge bath, don't fill the tub too much; have the child sit in 20 cm (eight inches) of water, leaving most of the body exposed to help evaporation. If the sponging makes the child feel chilled, shivery, or unhappy, it should be stopped. For safety reasons, children should never be left alone in the bathtub.

Are there non-prescription drugs that bring down fever?

If medication is used to relieve the discomfort associated with a child's fever, paracetamol is the drug of choice. It's not costly, it has few side-effects, and it's available in many forms for children, including drops, elixir (flavoured syrup), capsules and suppositories. Don't expect it to lower the child's

---

A word about ASA and aspirin

Acetylsalicylic acid is known generically as 'aspirin'.

Although asprin is effective in reducing fevers, it is *not generally recommended for sick children* because of its side-effects. In particular, it's associated with Reye's syndrome, a rare condition that causes swelling of the brain and serious illness, and can be fatal.

---

temperature to normal, but it should bring it down to a more comfortable level. The dose range recommended is 10 to 15 mg/kg (milligrams per kilo of body weight) administered every four hours when necessary. (Thus a child who weighs 20 kilos, would be given a dosage of 200 to 300 mg.) It has been shown that many parents use a much lower dose of paracetamol than the child's age or weight requires. It is perfectly safe and acceptable to use this drug at 15 mg/kg, and this dose is recommended by many doctors.

If the child vomits or spits up the medication immediately, or within 10 to 15 minutes, the entire dose may be given again. If the child can't tolerate the paracetamol by mouth, a suppository can be tried.

Ibuprofen, another medication used to treat fever and pain, is available as a liquid and as tablets. The dose of Ibuprofen is 5 to 10 mg/kg, given every six hours when needed. Ibuprofen should not be used for fever and pain in children with chickenpox and should be used with caution when children have poor fluid intake.

Remember that these medications are not cures, and should not be given automatically. If your feverish child is not uncomfortable, there is no need to bring the fever down.

Convulsions Due to Fever

Convulsions due to fever, or 'febrile seizures,' affect approximately one in 25 children who have a fever between the ages of six months and 4 to 5 years. The seizures are very upsetting, even terrifying, to parents, but they don't do any harm; the child won't die from the seizure and won't suffer any brain damage. Furthermore, studies show that 97 percent of all children with febrile seizures do not develop epilepsy, which is a different condition.

What happens in a febrile seizure?

During the seizure the child loses consciousness and stiffens, the lips turn blue, and the whole body may begin to jerk. When the convulsive movements stop, the child regains consciousness but may be sleepy and groggy for a while. The most important thing is to remain calm and not panic, however frightening the convulsion may appear. Place the child on a soft surface, lying on his or her side. Don't put anything in the child's mouth. The child will *not* choke or 'swallow' his or her tongue. The convulsion usually stops within a few minutes, without any medication. If it persists for more than 5 to 10 minutes, take the child to the nearest doctor or hospital; convulsions that last longer than 10 to 20 minutes may require medication to stop them. Calling an ambulance is safer than driving your child to hospital at high speed when you are distracted by anxiety.

Children outgrow the tendency to have febrile seizures by the time they're four or five, but some children have recurrences. Even recurrent febrile seizures are not harmful and do not result in brain damage, death, or epilepsy. Unfortunately there is no known way of preventing the seizures. Although paracetamol will lower the fever and make the child more comfortable, there is no evidence that it will prevent a seizure.

A child who has had a seizure associated with fever should be treated normally in all respects, and should resume normal activities. Being overprotective of a child just because there is a history of febrile seizures will only do harm.

CHAPTER 6

Toilet-Training

· ·

Toilet-training your child can be a real challenge. Some children master the skill with seemingly little effort on the part of their parents, while others need a great deal of encouragement. The processes of bladder and bowel control, which most of us take for granted, demand fairly sophisticated coordination.

How do children learn to control their bladders?

Significant changes occur in bladder control from birth through childhood. In the infant, before bladder control is achieved, emptying and filling are automatic. The infant's bladder only holds about 50 ccs (less than two ounces), so voiding cannot be delayed. Between the ages of one and two, as the brain matures, the infant becomes aware of the sensation of a full bladder and the need to urinate. In addition, bladder capacity increases so that the bladder doesn't have to empty as frequently. With further maturing, the child develops the ability to control the external sphincter muscle voluntarily, postponing urination until a toilet is available, even though the bladder is full. Daytime dryness is thus achieved.

How do children learn bowel control?

In infants, although the frequency and consistency of stool vary, depending on the diet, an individual pattern of stooling develops for each child and should not require parental intervention. Later, usually between two and three years of age, the child learns to recognise fullness of the lower large bowel as the sign that stooling is imminent, and to indicate that need. At first, this warning gives the parent a little time to supply a potty or toilet. Later,

Bladder control

Two ureters carry urine from the kidneys to the bladder, a hollow structure surrounded by a muscular wall that relaxes when urine is being stored. When the muscle contracts, increasing the pressure in the bladder, and the bladder opening relaxes, the result is voiding of urine (urination). The urine then passes through the urethra and outside the body.

Two sphincters (muscular mechanisms) control the bladder. One is the inner sphincter at the bladder neck or outlet; stimulation of this muscle holds the urethra closed, keeping urine in the bladder, and relaxation allows voiding down the urethra. This mechanism is not under voluntary control. The other, the external sphincter, close to the outside end of the urethra, is under voluntary control. Stimulation of this muscle keeps the urethra closed and holds urine in the bladder; relaxation is essential for voiding.

Messages from the bladder to the brain (such as 'I'm full!'), and from the brain to the bladder (such as 'Hold on!') travel via the nerves of the spinal cord. These nerves are essential for the control of bladder function.

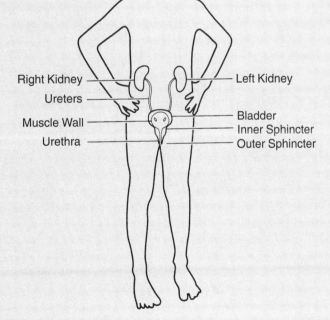

Right Kidney —   — Left Kidney
Ureters —
Muscle Wall —   — Bladder
Urethra —   — Inner Sphincter
   — Outer Sphincter

as the child gains more control over the external sphincter of the bowel, stooling can be delayed. But while a delay may be convenient, note that repeated or prolonged withholding can lead to problems with constipation, stretching and thinning of the bowel muscles, and even soiling (see below). A child who 'needs to poo' should be given the chance as soon as possible.

By the time they start to recognise that stooling is imminent, most children have already stopped stooling into nappies at night. Daytime bladder control is usually achieved next, followed by daytime bowel control.

Bowel control

The nutrients from our food are absorbed into the bloodstream from the part of the bowel called the small intestine. After passing through this part of the bowel, any remaining contents enter the large intestine, which is responsible for further absorption of water and formation of the final stool. The wall of the large intestine is composed of muscle fibres and nerves. The muscle propels the waste products towards the anal opening, and the nerves carry messages between the muscle and the brain.

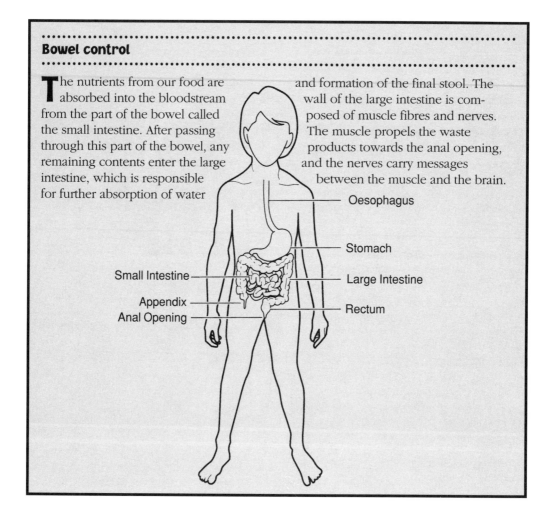

- Oesophagus
- Stomach
Small Intestine
- Large Intestine
Appendix
Anal Opening
- Rectum

How will I know when my child is ready for toilet-training?

Children need to be ready both physically and temperamentally for this important event. Although it's possible to predict the reflex emptying of an infant's bladder or bowel, and therefore to be lucky enough to catch the urine or stool in a vessel, this is not the same as the infant mastering bladder and bowel control. In deciding when to begin real toilet-training, you should consider several factors.

Often children begin to imitate siblings or parents, and to show an interest in the passage of urine and stool from their bodies and the use of potties or toilets. Signals that the child is aware of a full bladder or bowel may be facial expressions, wriggling movements, or other signs that parents usually interpret quickly and correctly. This is an important first step in toilet-training. The bladder should have matured to the point that your child is able to stay dry for several hours and pass a reasonable quantity of urine at each voiding. The desire for independence and increasing competence will lead your child to an interest in managing toiletting, and allowing the child to progress at his or her own pace, without conflict and tension, is thought to be important.

It's reasonable to start training when your child is able to walk, to get to the potty or toilet without help. The combination of understanding the purpose of the toilet, being aware of the need to urinate or stool, and feeling displeasure at being wet or dirty is important in the process. If these milestones coincide with the child's desire to please you by mastering the skills *before* the child reaches the phase of saying no to everything, toilet-training can often be easily achieved. Consequently you should try to be sensitive to your child's development, provide opportunities for mastering toiletting skills without coercion, and postpone the process if the child shows resistance.

What's the best approach to toilet-training?

There's a wide variety of cultural influences on toilet-training methods, and your family and cultural expectations should be respected and integrated into your method of toilet-training, and indeed into all aspects of child-rearing. There are no good studies to tell us which method of toilet-training is the most successful. However, some suggestions have been accepted as 'good advice.'

The use of a potty as an introduction to the toilet is favoured by many. The potty has the advantages of being a more appropriate size for a young child, being closer to the floor, and allowing the child's feet to remain on the floor; it's also portable. Some children express a fear of the toilet, imagining that monsters will 'nip their bums' or that they'll fall in and be flushed away. This fear can be minimised by simple reassurance and by providing adaptable seating and a bench under the feet. Appropriate posture, with the hips and knees at right angles and the feet against a firm surface, may make defecation easier. Be sure to allow the child enough time for complete urination or defecation, and to encourage successful completion, as this will build up the child's sense of accomplishment.

Young children need help in using the toilet for a while, but as they get better at dressing and undressing they learn to manage visits on their own. Accidents may still occur in the daytime, as a child can delay urination only a few minutes after feeling the initial urge. As the child matures, these accidents become less frequent. If a child at any time becomes difficult to handle or resists toiletting regularly, it's usually better to stop your efforts for a few months and then start again. Children usually learn quickly when they are ready.

 ### What about night-time?

Bowel emptying at night has usually stopped before daytime bowel training begins. However, night wetting usually persists after daytime dryness has been achieved. There is no clear evidence whether the method and timing of toilet-training accelerate or retard night-time dryness. When your child has achieved reasonable control in the day, the nappies can be left off except at night. When he or she is dry on wakening, night-time dryness has been achieved and the nappies can be abandoned.

 ### What about children who keep on wetting?

Most normal children achieve daytime dryness by age four and night-time dryness by age five, though boys tend to be later than girls. Persistence of wetting beyond these ages is referred to as 'daytime (diurnal) enuresis' and 'night-time (nocturnal) enuresis' – also known as 'bedwetting.' Daytime and night-time wetting may both be present. If the child has been dry for a minimum of six months and then has an onset of wetting, day or night, it's called 'secondary.' If such a dry period has never occurred, the wetting is 'primary.'

Daytime wetting occurs in about one percent of children aged 7 to 12. But 15 percent of children are still wetting the bed at night at age five. As they mature, some of them outgrow the problem; only five percent of ten-year-olds, two percent of 16-year-olds, and fewer than one percent of adults have this problem. The factors that contribute to night-time wetting beyond the age of five are a delay in the maturing of the mechanisms required for bladder control, and an inherited predisposition. If both parents were bedwetters, there is a 77 percent chance of their child being a bedwetter. If one parent was a bedwetter, there is a 44 percent chance.

Your child's mastery of bladder control should be discussed at your regular visits to the child's doctor. You can express your concerns about any delays, and seek advice on maintaining a reasonable plan for toilet-training. If unusual urinary symptoms develop, such as frequency of urination or pain on urination, arrange for assessment by a doctor. Persistence of wetting beyond the expected age should also trigger a further assessment.

 How will the doctor make this assessment?

The doctor will take a history of many aspects of the child's problem. It will be important to know whether the accidents are happening in the daytime or night-time, or both, and whether the wetting is primary or secondary. The doctor will ask if there are any associated symptoms, such as pain on urination, that might suggest a urinary-tract infection. A history of the child's toilet-training is helpful in understanding daytime difficulties in particular, while a history of the child's general health and development lets the doctor consider any other medical or developmental problems that might explain the delay in bladder control. The doctor may also ask if you are concerned about any other behavioural problems that might reflect the maturity or compliance of the child, or any fears the child may have. For example, fear of the dark can make it difficult for a child to leave their bed at night to go to the bathroom. It's also helpful to know what treatments have been tried so far.

A family history, particularly of the parents, is useful to determine if either parent was a bedwetter. If there is any family history of kidney disease, you may be anxious to rule out the possibility of kidney disease in your child.

The doctor will also explore the emotional aspects of the wetting. How does the child cope? How is the child's self-esteem? What does the wetting prevent the child from doing? For example, does he or she miss sleep-overs with friends, or going to camp? What is the attitude of the family towards the bedwetting? Is either parent upset, angry, or frustrated? How have the parents responded to each bedwetting episode? Do they blame the child, or each other?

The doctor will then do a full examination, with particular attention to the abdomen, the spine, the genitalia, and the nerves that supply the organs that control urination.

For children who have night-time wetting as their only problem, a urine test is usually enough to rule out urine problems. If the child has daytime wetting, a urine test will still be appropriate, but it may be necessary to do other tests as well, depending on what the doctor finds.

 ### Why do some children have 'accidents' after they are toilet-trained?

The child may be too busy playing to answer the body's signals that the bladder is full, or may have suppressed the urge on several occasions, until the need to urinate became overwhelming and the child couldn't make it to the bathroom in time. It's important to watch for signals of your child's desire to urinate, and especially for signals that he or she is trying to suppress the urge – for example, squatting, pressing a heel into the genital area, dancing around, or crossing the legs. You should encourage your child to empty his or her bladder when the 'need to go' signal occurs; that habit plays an important role in the mastery of urinary habits.

Sometimes stress is involved; the hospitalisation of a young child, separation from parents, or a family break-up may make a child regress to wetting. The recurrence of daytime wetting may also signal the onset of a medical problem such as a urinary-tract infection, so a doctor's advice should be sought. Other symptoms of urinary-tract infections may include frequency of urination, altered smell and colour of the urine, and possibly fever and lower-abdominal pain. A urine test will be required to rule out the possibility of infection. Once the problem has been dealt with, retraining in toilet habits may be required.

 ### Why do some children keep on bedwetting?

Parents often note that their bedwetting child is a deep sleeper. Sleep studies have failed to show that bedwetting is associated with a particular stage of sleep; however, there is some evidence that arousal times are different for bedwetters than for children who have night-time control of urination. Perhaps it just takes these children too long to wake up. There is no evidence that small bladder capacity, serious psychological disorder, or allergic problems are responsible for most cases of bedwetting. Physical abnormalities occasionally cause the persistence or onset of night-time wetting beyond five years of age, but that possibility can be checked by the doctor.

 ### What can I do about a bedwetter?

You can start by explaining the likely cause of the problem to your child, clearly and in age-appropriate language. In most cases this means explaining that the tendency is inherited and developmental, and outside the child's control, and that it's not any kind of illness. Have an open discussion of other causes the child may have heard you blame, and reassure him or her that no one thinks the problem is rooted in laziness.

As for practical measures, once it's clear that the child has no underlying kidney problems, supportive measures should be adopted. Some families choose to live with the problem, and manage it by using plastic sheets on the bed and changing the sheets immediately after a wetting episode, or in the morning if the child has not awakened. There are mattress covers available that absorb the majority of the wetness and can be placed immediately underneath where the child sleeps. Sometimes children are encouraged to participate in stripping the bed; this is appropriate as long as it's done to encourage self-sufficiency, and not in a punitive fashion. Some parents say that encouraging the child to wear pull-up nappies of an appropriate size is helpful. Most children over the age of six find this babyish and unacceptable, but the strategy may be useful for overnight trips. The child can often manage such nappies on his or her own, if easy disposal is available; failing that, send along a plastic bag to ensure safe transportation home.

A few children develop skin irritation and rashes secondary to the wetness, but the vast majority do not. If a rash does develop, changing the wet clothing as soon as urination occurs is an important preventive measure, and barrier creams will help prevent the rash from getting worse.

 Would it help if I limited my child's fluid intake after supper?
This simple manoeuvre is successful in some children, but certainly not in all. It makes sense that drinking large quantities of liquid before bedtime will challenge any bladder during the night hours. However, normal amounts of fluid should be allowed and no child should be made to go to bed thirsty.

 What about waking the child up for a bathroom trip before I go to bed myself?
Some parents find that rousing the child to go to the bathroom at their bedtime prevents further wetting during the night. However, many children don't wake up enough at this time to make themselves urinate. If the strategy works for your child, by all means use it. However, it is not appropriate to disturb your own night's sleep with repeated awakenings to rouse the child.

 Should I try some sort of reward system?
You might try putting up a big calendar and letting your child keep a record

of dry nights and wet nights. A dry night earns the child a sticker or gold star, and some further reward if you want. This method of rewarding dry nights has been shown to be successful in approximately 20 percent of children, so it's worth trying as a first-line measure. Unfortunately, some children relapse and are unable to maintain dryness in spite of the rewards.

 ### Do bedwetting alarms work?

The most commonly used bedwetting alarm consists of a battery-operated machine; a device for sensing wetness, which is attached to the child's underwear or pyjamas, close to the urethral opening; and a buzzer attached to the child's clothing on the shoulder, close to the ear. The first few drops of urine passed should touch the sensor and set off the alarm, which should waken the child, and thus stop the urination. The child then disconnects the alarm and gets up to go to the bathroom. If the child has more than one wet episode in a night, the underwear should be changed and the alarm reset to catch the next bedwetting episode. This method is the most successful form of treatment available and works for 70 to 90 percent of children. However, the child must be mature enough, developmentally and emotionally, and motivated enough to deal with the signals. Although you can come and attempt to assist the child in waking up, perhaps by placing a wet cloth on his or her forehead, it's essentially the child who must respond to the alarm. As this is a training regimen, be prepared to try the alarm for at least a month, and probably two. Although 20 percent of children relapse when they stop using the alarm, the majority remain dry.

The alarm system is less likely to work for a child of six or seven, and more likely to work for the child of nine or older, particularly one who is very highly motivated to achieve dryness. A calendar is kept during the period of treatment to record wet and dry nights, as well as 'damp only' episodes when the alarm roused the child enough to pass most of the urine in the toilet. It's interesting that children who achieve dryness from this treatment don't necessarily wake up at night to pass their urine, but are able to sleep through the night. Presumably their bodies learn to hold urine in spite of the bladder being full. The alarm systems cost around $60 and have replaceable batteries. One supplier of a commonly used alarm (Dri Sleeper) can be found at www.dri-sleeper.com (Alpha consultants, PO Box 569, Nelson, Ph 03 548 9592). Of course, they don't work for deaf children, and they may not be suitable for children who sleep with siblings or parents, or those who are too fearful of the noise to use the alarm successfully.

There are older alarm systems that are placed under the bedsheets, but they are less successful as more urine needs to be passed before the alarm goes off. A new alarm with a vibrating signal has recently become available, but there are as yet no studies to document its effectiveness.

I've heard of something called 'Azrin's system' – what's that?

This multidimensional approach to bedwetting uses several techniques to reinforce dryness, including night-time wakening, positive and negative reinforcement, bladder-control training, and the use of a urine alarm. The alarm is a proven form of therapy, but the addition of the other components has not clearly been shown to be useful.

Do bladder-control exercises do any good?

Some (not all) children with bedwetting may have a smaller functional bladder capacity than normal for their age. Bladder-training exercises have been attempted, to encourage children to hold urine a few minutes beyond their initial urge to urinate. Studies are inconclusive as to whether these exercises make a difference to the frequency of bedwetting.

Aren't there any medications that help?

Several medications have been shown to be of benefit in treating bedwetting. However, it's essential to look at the harm a medication may do, as well as its success, since bedwetting is a developmental condition that will eventually go away on its own.

Imipramine (Tofranil) was originally introduced as an antidepressant but was found to be successful in reducing bedwetting episodes. It's effective in only about half the children who try it, and its side-effects include emotional instability, sleep disturbances, lethargy, dry mouth, and mild stomach upsets, to name a few. However, many children tolerate the medicine without any difficulty. Note that imipramine is a *very dangerous drug* when too much is taken; overdoses can lead to heart and breathing problems, convulsions, and even death. Be sure to keep it locked away from children, except for the prescribed dose.

More recently, desmopressin acetate (DDAVP) has been introduced for the treatment of bedwetting. This is a different form of a naturally occurring substance called 'antidiuretic hormone,' which helps the body retain water and prevents its excretion. It has been suggested that bedwetting children suffer from decreased levels of antidiuretic hormone, or do not respond normally to it. Although this has not been proven conclusively, DDAVP decreases bedwetting in approximately half of children. It is administered by nasal spray, in a dosage of 1 to 4 puffs (10 to 40 micrograms), before going to bed. It may not work if the child has a cold or allergic nasal inflammation, as this can interfere with its absorption. Its side-effects include irritation of the nose and eyes, but it is usually well tolerated. It does have a very low risk of causing significant disturbances in the body's fluid and salt composition, which can lead to convulsions, so whenever the child is sick with vomiting and diarrhoea the drug should be discontinued. Also, caution the child against drinking unnecessary excess fluid while on the medication. DDAVP can be very useful for ensuring dryness on overnight stays with friends or during attendance at camp. The benefit usually ceases when the medication is stopped.

Oxybutynin (Ditropan) has not been proven useful in night-time wetting, but has been used successfully to help improve bladder capacity in some children with daytime wetting.

What about non-drug therapies?
Some parents have found hypnotherapy helpful in getting their children to stop bedwetting. However, this remains a controversial area and there is no clear evidence to support its use.

Rarely, emotional disturbances are involved in bedwetting. In such cases, psychotherapy may help; stresses can be discussed, and appropriate support mechanisms put in place. However, there is no role for psychotherapy in the treatment of most bedwetting children.

What about a child who defecates in the wrong place?
This is called 'soiling' – the repeated voluntary or involuntary passage of stools in inappropriate places, such as into underwear or onto the floor. Most children have achieved bowel control by age four if they have otherwise normal development. Persistence of soiling beyond that age is referred to as 'primary' soiling, or encopresis. If the child has had a minimum of six months without soiling and then begins to soil, this is called 'secondary' encopresis. Unfortunately, soiling leaves an offensive odour, so the child may be ridiculed and isolated. There is often friction within the family, and the child may be the target of anger and blame.

What makes a child soil?

The most common cause is constipation. Retention of stools leads to stretching of the large bowel wall, which leads to a decrease in its ability to contract and propel the contents forward. More water is absorbed from the stool because it stays longer in the large bowel, and so larger and harder stools are formed. The passage of these stools is often painful, and may even cause stretching and tearing of the anal opening (fissures); as a result, the child may delay stooling, which makes the problem even worse. There are also some children who have incomplete emptying of the bowel; they seem to have 'regular' bowel movements but in fact retain considerable amounts of stool. In either case, the retained stool can form 'rocks,' and then softer stool may leak around these, resulting in soiling.

Several factors are believed to contribute to the development of this problem. In infancy, constipation, abnormalities of the lower bowel (anus and rectum), and forceful interventions by parents may set the scene for later development of soiling. In the toddler and preschool years, painful or difficult stooling (for a variety of reasons), forceful toilet-training, psychosocial stresses that interfere with toilet-training, or unusual fear of the toilet may contribute further to the risk. As the child passes into school age, other risk factors emerge: avoidance of school toilets, difficulties with staying at tasks (attention deficit), busy family lifestyles, and similar psychosocial stresses. Many children cope with these stresses, but some, especially those with several risk factors, go on to develop soiling.

Constipation is not always involved; diarrhoea may also lead to loss of control over stool. Acute infections or gastroenteritis in a young child may result in temporary soiling. However, this usually resolves itself. Repeated episodes of loose stool that can't be traced to underlying medical problems are probably more akin to 'irritable bowel syndrome' in adults.

There is also a small group of children who have 'manipulative' soiling, which is not caused by constipation, though constipation may be present. These children appear to be expressing strong feelings (anger or sadness) through their bowels.

Rarely, a medical problem lies behind the soiling.

What can I do if my child is soiling?

It's very important to get a full medical assessment: a history of bowel habits, toilet-training, other developmental and health issues, family history, and stresses on the child, followed by a complete physical examination.

Special tests are occasionally done to clarify or rule out medical causes for the problem.

The treatment will depend on the cause or the factors contributing to the soiling. Any constipation can be managed by a regimen of altered diet and improved bowel habits to empty the bowel of retained stool and encourage the passage of smaller, softer stools. Stool softeners or other laxatives may also be recommended. Careful attention to regular toilet visits, provision of adequate time for stooling, and rewarding of appropriate stooling behaviour are critical. If serious underlying stresses or problems exist, more specific therapy will be required.

CHAPTER 7

Spilling, Vomiting, and Diarrhoea

● ●

Spilling and regurgitation often occur in early infancy, and are usually related to feeding. The difference between spilling, regurgitation, and vomiting is often not clear, and these symptoms may seem to merge into one another at times. Many infants have them to varying degrees in the first few months of life.

Q What's the difference between 'spilling' and 'regurgitation'?

Many babies voluntarily expel milk while they're feeding, pushing the liquid out of their mouths with their tongues. The amount of breast milk or formula lost this way is small, and simple 'spilling' by itself is never associated with significant disease unless an infant fails to gain weight and thrive. At times babies spill simply because they've taken in too much milk, or because a bubble of air is escaping the stomach.

Spilling is not a good reason to change a child's formula. It's a benign condition that usually improves by six months of age and resolves itself by 8 to 12 months of age.

Regurgitation is also common in early infancy, but it can be an indication of serious gastrointestinal illness at this age. Regurgitation is the effortless expulsion of the contents of the stomach; the amount of regurgitated food varies and may or may not be significant. This symptom may occur at any time, with the infant in any position, but it's most common immediately after the child has eaten. Usually liquid and solid foods are regurgitated equally. If regurgitation persists, it should be evaluated by your child's general practitioner, who will want to know how soon after birth you noticed the baby regurgitating, and whether the fluid that is regurgitated is bile (yellow) or blood stained. The presence of bile or blood may be an indication of serious disease and you should consult your general practitioner immediately. Most important, the doctor will check whether your child has gained enough weight since the regurgitation began. If the weight gain has been normal, there is likely very little to be concerned about. The doctor will also want to know if the child is choking during the episodes of regurgitation, and if the child's lips turn blue or he or she seems to stop breathing momentarily. These symptoms are more serious indications of illness. There are several gastrointestinal conditions associated with persistent regurgitation in childhood, but the most common is gastroesophageal reflux (GOR). Premature infants are very likely to have GOR.

 ### What exactly is GOR?

In GOR, the valve at the lower end of the oesophagus, leading to the stomach, is not as tight as normal. In the first 8 to 12 weeks of life, all children have some looseness of this valve. Between three and nine months of age, the valve tightens and the reflux (regurgitation) becomes less frequent. No treatment is necessary unless the episodes of reflux are accompanied by 'blue spells' – episodes where breathing seems temporarily stopped – or the infant is not gaining weight. In a more severely affected infant, repositioning the child after feeding, changing feeding routines, and thickening the feeds may reduce the reflux.

Persistent severe GOR may be associated with weight loss and chronic irritability. The irritability is the result of stomach acid and partially digested food flowing back into the lower esophagus. In extreme cases the irritation causes bleeding, and anaemia may result. If the situation continues unchecked for a long time, the lower esophagus may narrow and require surgical treatment. Severe GOR can also be responsible for recurrent coughing and wheezing episodes in infancy, due to stomach contents entering the back of the throat and the lungs.

 ### Can allergies cause regurgitation?

Regurgitation is caused by a child's allergy to cow's milk or to other foods in about 20 percent of cases. Some infants are changed from cow's-milk formula to an alternative formula to relieve the problem. If an infant has a history of chronic sniffles or a clear nasal discharge that defies explanation, has other allergic reactions such as eczema, or has a strong family background of food allergy, then allergy may be considered as a cause.

What's the difference between regurgitation and vomiting?

Vomiting is the *forceful* expulsion of stomach contents. It's a more serious symptom than spilling or regurgitation, and can lead to significant medical problems if it persists. In older children who don't appear severely ill, vomiting may disappear without treatment within 12 to 24 hours, but a young infant or child who is vomiting needs to be assessed sooner because of the risk of dehydration. Vomiting can be associated with minor illnesses, but it can also be the first symptom of more serious problems, such as intestinal obstruction, inflammation, or meningitis. That's why it's important to tell the doctor when a young child – especially an infant – is vomiting.

That doesn't mean that all vomiting is serious. A child who is suddenly frightened may vomit, as may a child who is angry, upset, or just very excited. Sometimes children vomit simply because they've gobbled up too much of a favourite food.

When you report vomiting to your child's doctor, you can help by having an accurate description of your child's condition in your mind. Does the child appear unwell? How long has the symptom been present? Is there a fever? If so, how high is it? Are there symptoms such as headache, neck pain, abdominal pain, diarrhoea, rash, earache, cough, or sore throat? Is the child producing urine in the usual amount? Is the material being vomited bile-stained (yellow or green) or blood-tinged? Can the child keep down *any* food or fluid? Do specific foods seem to cause the problem? Has the child taken any medication that might provoke vomiting as a side-effect, or come in contact with spoiled food? Is anyone else in the house ill? Could the child have accidentally got into any medication or household products? From the answers to these questions your doctor can decide whether the child can be managed at home, needs to be seen in the surgery, or needs prompt referral to your local emergency department.

When vomiting needs immediate attention

A child with bile-stained or bloody vomitus, who is vomiting frequently and has a distended, swollen abdomen and severe abdominal pain accompanied by lethargy and irritability, is in urgent need of medical attention. A young child who has been vomiting longer than 12 to 24 hours, is unable to hold down any fluids, and has reduced urinary output should be assessed by a doctor.

What are the more serious causes of vomiting?

In the period shortly after birth, vomiting can be due to obstruction of the gastrointestinal tract. The most common reason for this is a muscular obstruction to the outflow valve of the stomach, called 'pyloric stenosis.' The condition is typically seen in newborns about 5 to 6 weeks of age, but may begin as early as 2 to 4 weeks of age. The vomiting is very forceful (projectile) and worsens as time goes on. The condition is more common in boys than in girls, and tends to run in families.

Infection of the urinary tract and *meningitis* are two serious conditions that may first appear as vomiting in early infancy. Meningitis is caused by bacteria inflaming the tissues around the brain (meninges). It is associated with fever, headache, neck stiffness, and extreme irritability. If not diagnosed and treated early, it leads to drowsiness, coma, and possible permanent brain damage or death. Significant fever along with vomiting in an infant who is feeding poorly and appears unwell should alert you to these possibilities.

Gastroesophageal reflux (GOR) is an important cause of vomiting in an infant, as noted above. Infants who have severe GOR may regurgitate their food and vomit as well. In severely affected infants, the vomiting may be blood-tinged. Typically, such infants are poor eaters and fail to thrive.

Coeliac disease is a rare condition caused by an inborn inability of the intestinal lining to handle gluten, a protein found in wheat. The resultant inflammation causes diarrhoea and the inability of the intestine to absorb necessary nutrients. What usually brings these children to the doctor is chronic diarrhoea and poor weight gain. Children with coeliac disease who are given a gluten-free diet do extremely well.

Rumination, the regurgitation of both liquid and solid food in a purposeful manner, can occur during feedings but is more common after a meal is completed. It can occur in any situation but is more common in children who are mentally handicapped or have significant mental illness. GOR can be associated with rumination.

Intestinal infection is another common cause of vomiting in infants and toddlers. Usually fever and diarrhoea are also present. Viral infections account for the vast majority of these illnesses, but about 20 percent are caused by bacterial infections. Often the stool contains blood. The high fever associated with these infections may lead to a febrile convulsion.

Intussusception is a serious but uncommon problem that occurs in infants and toddlers, in which one section of intestine 'folds' inside another. The onset of attacks of severe abdominal pain in a previously healthy child, accompanied by vomiting and the eventual appearance (in most cases) of a red jelly-like stool (blood), suggests this condition. Early diagnosis of intussusception leads to successful treatment. Fortunately, the other causes of intestinal obstruction in childhood are quite rare.

Inflammation of the appendix is the commonest reason for abdominal surgery in childhood. Although abdominal pain is the main symptom, vomiting commonly accompanies the pain. This condition is unusual in infants and toddlers; it's much more likely to occur in older children and adolescents. The appendix, a small piece of intestine that serves no useful role, may get obstructed and inflamed. Abdominal pain and fever, with vomiting and no diarrhoea, should prompt you to have your child checked for appendicitis. If your child has this problem, surgery to remove the inflamed appendix is necessary and solves the problem forever.

Neurological conditions can also cause vomiting in children. A head injury, with or without loss of consciousness, must be monitored closely if the child begins to vomit. Migraine headaches can also be accompanied by vomiting. Although brain tumours are infrequent in childhood, the presence of a persistent headache accompanied by vomiting in a child who does not feel nauseated and does not have a fever must be brought to the attention of the child's doctor.

Vomiting may also be associated with heavy bouts of coughing. For example, whooping cough is frequently associated with vomiting, and so is asthma.

How can I stop my child's vomiting?

Fortunately, most children stop vomiting without any medical treatment. It's important to position a vomiting child on his or her side so that vomited material won't be breathed into the lungs. Children who vomit continuously and are unable to keep any liquids down, or who have diarrhoea and fever, must be watched closely for dehydration.

Are there medications that stop vomiting?

It's extremely important *not* to use over-the-counter remedies for childhood vomiting without consulting your doctor. Some medications can mask a child's symptoms, or prevent you from making an accurate assessment of your child's progress. Few, if any, of these remedies are truly effective in controlling the cause of vomiting.

71

The risks of dehydration

When the body loses large quantities of water, through vomiting, diarrhoea, or even just sweating, it also loses essential minerals called 'electrolytes.' Without enough water and electrolytes, the body's functioning can be seriously impaired. Dehydration is potentially life-threatening, and requires early recognition and treatment.

Dehydration can be recognised by lack of moisture in mucous membranes; look for a dry mouth, no saliva production, an absence of tears, weight loss, lethargy and irritability, and decreased urine output. The urine may be abnormally dark in colour, because waste products are less diluted with water.

Dehydration can be treated by restoring the lost fluids and electrolytes. Studies have shown that early use of an oral electrolyte solution (such as Pedialyte) is the best treatment.

If a child has been vomiting, it's a good idea to wait an hour after the last episode before attempting rehydration. Then give a small volume of oral electrolyte solution – 60 to 90 ml (two or three ounces) – every 30 to 40 minutes, until the child seems stable enough to accept plain foods. Occasionally, children who don't respond to oral electrolyte solution need to be hospitalised and given fluids through a nasogastric tube or intravenous drip.

If the child is dehydrated, use an oral electrolyte solution to combat the dehydration. Once the child has kept down the solution for several hours without significant vomiting, simple solids – bread, crackers, pasta, potatoes – can be reintroduced into the diet. A breast-feeding infant can have breast milk. If these foods are well tolerated, the child can return to a normal diet. A child who can't hold down oral replacement fluids or simple solid foods in the first 12 to 24 hours should be assessed by a doctor.

Diarrhoea

The normal pattern of bowel movements varies in consistency and frequency, depending on the child's age and the composition of the diet. In the newborn period, babies who are breast-fed may have up to 10 small bowel movements per day, often one after each feeding. The normal stool of a breast-fed infant has a pasty consistency and a mustard-like colour. By the end of the twelfth week, the frequency of the infant's stool has decreased. Some infants begin to have semifirm stool once daily or every other day. By the age of 18 to 30 months, most children have one or two formed bowel movements each day.

As a parent, you become accustomed to the consistency, amount, and frequency of your infant's bowel movements. Suddenly they may become loose, and increase in volume and frequency. The colour may change, and a foul odour may be evident when the stools are passed. This is diarrhoea.

Is diarrhoea serious?

An occasional loose stool is no cause for alarm. Most often, diarrhoea is mild and clears up without treatment in one or two days. However, if the symptom is accompanied by high fever, if your child appears ill, and if he or she has copious quantities of explosive movements, with or without vomiting, consult the doctor.

Diarrhoea or loose bowel movements can be caused by simple overfeeding. In this case the stools are semiformed and can be frequent, but are seldom discoloured or malodorous. A child should never be forced to take more milk than he or she seems to want.

Many parents of young toddlers are concerned by the presence of undigested food particles in the child's loose stool. This finding is not abnormal, and means little in terms of diagnosis.

The sudden onset of loose, watery bowel movements along with increased stool volume may be a more serious sign, especially if the child is vomiting and feverish. Severe diarrhoea, especially in young infants, merits a call to the doctor, as well as close observation of the child because of the risk of dehydration.

What else causes diarrhoea?

Diarrhoea can be a side-effect of medication, especially certain antibiotics. If your child has unexpected diarrhoea and is taking medications, check with your doctor.

When a breast-fed infant develops diarrhoea, the mother may continue to breast-feed as long as the child's symptoms remain mild. If the infant is otherwise well, look for recent changes in the mother's diet, or any new medication the mother may be taking; either one may possibly be affecting the baby. Other non-infectious causes of diarrhoea include acute poisoning with iron, lead, mercury, or fluoride; food poisoning; and intussusception (see page 70).

When the lining of a child's intestine is damaged because of infection, diarrhoea is the result. The damaged lining can no longer digest or absorb foods normally, and the lack of complete digestion and absorption is complicated by the fact that the damaged bowel lining can secrete minerals and fluid into the intestine. Until recently, feeding the child liquids flavoured with large amounts of sugar was a common recommendation. In fact this can make diarrhoea *worse*; the build-up of unabsorbed sugar may cause the body to secrete more water into the intestine, making the stools even more watery.

'Enteritis' is inflammation or damage of the intestinal wall. When the lining of the stomach is also inflamed or damaged, the condition is called 'gastroenteritis.' In children, the commonest cause of acute diarrhoea is enteritis brought on by a virus. Fever may be present, as may vomiting. The bowel movements of children with viral gastroenteritis are greenish and very liquid. On occasion it may be difficult to distinguish them from urine in the nappy. If the stools look bloody or are black in appearance, there may be bleeding from the bowel lining. Blood in the stools can be associated with viral diarrhoea, but more commonly indicates bacterial enteritis. In any case, bloody stools should be reported to a doctor. Bacterial enteritis may also be accompanied by severe, crampy abdominal pains.

Children with acute infectious diarrhoea are contagious and may require a short period of isolation.

What about children with chronic diarrhoea?

Chronic diarrhoea can also be of infectious origin. Parasites such as *Giardia* and *Dientamoeba fragilis* are common in daycare populations (affecting 10 to 15 percent of children), though many children carrying these parasites have no symptoms. Non-infectious causes of chronic diarrhoea include ulcerative colitis, Crohn's disease, lactase deficiency, malabsorption, cystic fibrosis, coeliac disease, disaccharidase deficiency, Hirschsprung's disease, and food allergy. Diarrhoea that lasts more than 3 to 4 days with no sign of improvement should be reported to your child's doctor, even if the child seems well otherwise.

Drinking too much fruit juice is a common cause of chronic diarrhoea in toddlers, and promptly ceases when the fruit juice is discontinued. The high concentration of sugar causes excess fluid to be poured into the intestine. Diluting the fruit juice half and half with water should lead to an improvement in the diarrhoea if this is the cause.

How is acute diarrhoea treated?

The treatment of acute diarrhoea of an infectious origin in non-hospitalised children is always controversial. The goal is to correct any fluid loss, as well as any electrolyte imbalance, and at the same time provide adequate nutrition.

Antibiotics do not help acute viral diarrhoea, but can be used to treat certain types of bacterial diarrhoea and the diarrhoea caused by certain parasites.

Diarrhoea medicines that can be obtained without prescription are not advisable for children. These agents do not repair the injury to the intestinal wall, and may actually make things worse by masking the symptoms and persuading you to feed your child before the child has recovered enough. The process causing the diarrhoea may worsen, with continuing losses of salt and water, while you may feel that your child is better because you see less diarrhoea.

The course of action currently recommended when your child has acute diarrhoea is to give an oral electrolyte solution (see above) in the first 24 hours. For breast-feeding infants, breast milk should be continued. Once the diarrhoea slows down (usually within 24 hours), the child can receive age-appropriate solid foods, followed by milk or formula. Solids include complex carbohydrates for older children – bread, pasta, rice, potato – and apple-sauce, bananas, and cereals containing rice for infants. Fluid in doses of 30 ml (2 tablespoons) per half-hour is suggested; gradually increase the amount as the child tolerates more.

In the case of prolonged or severe diarrhoea, milk or formula low in lactose may be necessary for a short period, until the bowel has repaired itself. Boiled skim milk should never be used to treat diarrhoea (or even given to normal children). Drink mixes and soft drinks are not ideal as they are low in electrolytes.

Call your doctor if the diarrhoea is increasing in amount despite treatment, especially if the child continues to have a fever and keeps vomiting. If the diarrhoea does not improve in 24 to 36 hours after oral-electrolyte treatment, or persists after 3 to 5 days, maintain close contact with your doctor.

CHAPTER 8

Painful Urination

Pain or discomfort on urination is a frequent complaint in children and adolescents, on its own or in combination with other complaints such as genital itching or pain, fever, difficulty urinating, and frequent urination. Infants and young children who can't complain in words may show signs of pain during urination by crying, drawing up their legs, and/or clutching at their genitals. Parents may notice changes in children's genitals (such as redness or swelling); changes in the smell or colour of the urine; vaginal discharge or bleeding; or abnormalities in the stream of urine, such as very frequent small urinations, or a weak, dribbling urine stream.

Fortunately, many of the minor changes parents notice are within the wide range of normal behaviour and urine characteristics, and don't indicate an illness or problem. For example, a young girl who complains of mild itching or burning during one episode of urination but not during subsequent urinations is likely to be perfectly well when assessed by a doctor. Similarly, parents may notice that their apparently healthy young boy is urinating more frequently and gets up once in the night to urinate after days when he's had large amounts of liquids, but not on other days. There are no simple guidelines that tell exactly when a minor change in urine habits means a real problem, but many doctors believe the following signs call for prompt medical advice:

- genital pain, swelling, discolouration, or tenderness;

- pain or burning during urination that is either persistent, or severe enough to cause crying or upset, or associated with fever;

- definite changes in the colour of urine, such as urine that appears pink, red, or 'cola' in colour;

- any changes in urination habits accompanied by abdominal or back pain, weight loss, appetite loss, vomiting, or lethargy.

  Signs that likely call for medical advice, though not so urgently, may include:

- mild burning, itching, or discomfort during urination that doesn't occur with every urination;

- minor changes in urination habits (increased frequency, new onset of getting up to urinate at night);

- persistent wetting of clothes during the day, or bedwetting (in a child who has been previously dry), which is not accompanied by pain or other signs of illness.

What causes painful urination?

There are many causes, and the significance depends very much on the age, sex, and circumstances of the child. The presence or absence of other complaints is often very important in helping to determine the cause and importance of the painful urination. The most common causes are vulvitis in girls, urinary-tract infection in boys and girls, and balanoposthitis in boys. 'Vulvitis' is irritation or infection of the sensitive, moist lining of the external female genitals, the vulva. 'Balanoposthitis' refers to irritation and/or infection of the sensitive moist lining of the tip of the penis and under the foreskin. Sometimes painful urination is clearly attributable to other causes, such as a bruise from an injury, a sexually transmitted infection, or passage of a urinary stone. Only very rarely do doctors have to consider causes such as a foreign object placed in the child's urethra (the tube that drains urine from the bladder), a partial blockage of the urethra, and so on.

How serious is a urinary-tract infection?

The term 'urinary-tract infection' refers to a bacterial infection of the urine and lining or organs of the urinary tract, the bladder, and/or the kidneys. The complaints associated with infected urine vary tremendously, and may be as mild and simple as burning with urination or as severe as fever, vomiting, abdominal pain, and lethargy. Since most such infections occur in children younger than three years of age, who may not be able to communicate pain on voiding, many infections are brought to the parents' attention by fever or other signs, rather than complaints of pain. It is not necessary to check the urine for infection every time a child has a fever, but infants less than six months old with fever, children with fever and abdominal pain or changes in urination, and children with fever but no obvious explanation such as a cough and runny nose should probably have their urine tested.

About urine tests

A urinary-tract infection is diagnosed when bacteria are found growing in urine obtained directly from the bladder. In older children, a sample is caught from the middle of a urine stream with a special sterile container, after the child's genitals have been gently washed and rinsed with clean water. This urine must be refrigerated immediately, and delivered to the laboratory as soon as possible. Urine caught in a non-sterile container, or in another way, such as with a urine bag stuck to the child's genital area, is likely to be contaminated, and may suggest an infection when none exists.

In younger children, where a mid-stream sample can't be obtained, a sample may have to be taken through special techniques such as introducing a very small, soft plastic tube (catheter) into the bladder through the urethra. While this may appear painful, it's often necessary in order to establish whether or not an infection exists. Since a urinary-tract infection may prompt several other actions, such as X-ray examinations – one of which may involve introducing a catheter into the bladder – it's clearly important to be certain about the diagnosis.

Children with bacterial infection of the urine can be roughly divided into three groups: those without any symptoms; those with inflammation and infection of the bladder; and those with inflammation and infection of the kidney. Young girls sometimes have bacterial growth in their urine without ever feeling unwell. In most cases this form of infection doesn't appear to cause any damage and doesn't require treatment, so there's no point doing a urine test on an apparently healthy child with no complaints of pain, fever, or urination problems. However, it's important to diagnose infections that cause these complaints and involve the bladder or kidneys. If they are left untreated or recur frequently, they may cause scarring and damage to the kidneys.

A simple abnormality called 'vesicoureteral reflux' may be found in up to a third of children with urinary-tract infection. Reflux means that some urine flushes back up to the kidneys when the bladder is emptied. This makes it more difficult for the body to keep the urine free from infection, so these children often have repeated urine infections. Reflux itself doesn't damage the kidneys or cause any complaints or symptoms. The vast majority of children with reflux live their lives with normal kidney function, and it's important not to give them unnecessary anxiety or a sense that they have kidney disease. However, those who have repeated or severe urine infections may end up with kidney injury, which sometimes results in problems such as high blood pressure. Other abnormalities of the kidneys or drainage system are also found, but these are rare.

Significant kidney injury following urinary-tract infections, with or without reflux, is extremely rare in children who are otherwise well. However, infants with urinary-tract infections, children with repeated infections, or children with other problems, such as poor growth or persistent problems with urinating, are probably at greater risk. These children may benefit from X-ray tests looking for abnormalities such as vesicoureteral reflux. It is not yet clear whether all children with their first urinary-tract infection benefit from these tests.

How are urinary-tract infections treated?

Children with proven urinary-tract infections that cause symptoms such as painful urination require antibiotics. In most cases these can be given by mouth, but young infants, or children with severe infection or problems such as vomiting, will require admission to hospital for antibiotic treatment. Children whose X-ray studies show abnormalities of the kidney drainage system, or who have repeated urine infections, appear to benefit from longer-term daily antibiotic treatment. This treatment – for six months or longer, depending on the problem – helps prevent repeat infections. Some children with urinary-tract infections have problems with frequent urination and daytime wetting that persist after treatment of the infection. Though many doctors suggest bladder-training exercises for these children (see Chapter 6, 'Toilet-Training'), no one knows whether these exercises prevent repeated infections.

What are the signs of vulvitis?

Vulvitis (or vulvovaginitis, when the vagina is also involved) can usually be seen on examination, as the vulva becomes red and sore to touch, and sometimes has a discharge. Aside from the itching and burning that often persist between urinations, and the discharge, vulvovaginitis does not involve other difficulties such as changes in urination habits or urine, fever, or other signs of illness.

Prior to puberty the surface of the vulva is thin and more susceptible to irritation and inflammation. Young girls often have brief recurrent episodes of vulvitis, apparently because irritants and moisture are trapped in the vulva. This is called 'non-specific' vulvitis. Sensitivity to soaps and perfumes, and the use of tight clothing or nappies that trap moisture, may account for some of the irritation. Some girls seem particularly prone to vulvitis during and following toilet-training; poor habits in cleaning the child's bottom may be part of the cause (see below).

Non-specific vulvitis is a concern mainly because of the discomfort it causes. However, over a period of time, chronic inflammation may cause changes such as labial agglutination, in which the *labia minora*, the thin flaps of tissue on either side of the urethral and vaginal openings, stick together. This may cause pain with urination, and the labia may bleed if attempts are made to pull them apart, but separation can usually be achieved with treatment.

Vulvitis may also be caused by a specific infection, such as group A streptococcus, the organism that causes 'strep throat,' or by a yeast called 'candida.' Pinworms, short thread-like parasitic worms that live in the intestines, may occasionally infect a young child and cause anal itching, burning, and/or vulvitis.

Once adolescent girls reach puberty, they appear less susceptible to irritants and moisture trapping, and are more likely to get the kinds of vulvovaginitis that occur in adult women. Perfumed sanitary pads, tampons, and other feminine-hygiene products may act as irritants for girls this age.

 ### How is vulvitis prevented and treated?

No particular routine has been tested or proven to work, but the following general steps are unlikely to cause harm, and experience suggests that they may prevent non-specific vulvitis, or promote healing.

- Use bath products carefully. Avoid bubble baths and perfumed bath or hygiene products, excessive use of shampoo or soap in the bathwater, and applying soap directly to the membranes of the vulva.

- Use frequent baths in plain, tepid water, followed by gentle drying, and give the vulval area a chance to air-dry after the bath. While the child still has discomfort, she may feel better having several baths a day, and may even be encouraged to urinate while sitting in the bath if urination causes significant pain.

- Select loose day and night clothing to promote circulation of air, and to prevent restriction and trapping of moisture and irritants.

- Carefully supervise toileting hygiene. Avoid contaminating the vulva with soiled toilet paper; always wipe from front to back, *away* from the vulva.

When vulvitis is severe, doesn't respond to simple measures, or is associated with a large amount of discharge (suggesting vulvovaginitis), the doctor will look for specific causes. The urine may be tested to ensure that no urinary-tract infection is present, and the child will be examined and perhaps given a few simple tests. If there are signs of vulvitis from germs such as group A streptococcus, candida, or pinworms, she will clearly benefit from antibiotics. However, if the bacteria found on the surface of the vulva are normally present in girls without vulvitis, antibiotics are unlikely to do any good. If your child has severe or long-lasting vulvitis and labial agglutination, an estrogen cream can be prescribed to assist in healing and separating the labia.

Girls with symptoms of vulvitis or vulvovaginitis who have engaged in sexual activity, or who may have been victims of sexual assault, require special assessment by a doctor familiar with these problems. In this case, pain with urination or vulvitis requires a diligent approach that includes a search for sexually transmitted infections such as chlamydia and gonorrhoea, as well as counselling for prevention of pregnancy and sexually transmitted diseases (including AIDS and hepatitis).

What about the problems boys have?

Uncircumcised boys occasionally develop inflammation of the membranes of the foreskin and the tip of the penis (the glans) covered by the foreskin. This is called 'balanoposthitis,' and it usually causes pain and swelling of the tip of the penis, in addition to painful urination. In some cases this condition appears without any obvious cause. If there is white or grey discharge from under the foreskin, the inflammation is due to infection. Sometimes attempts to force back a foreskin that doesn't retract easily irritate the membranes and cause painful urination – or a painful swollen glans and difficult or painful urination can be caused when a foreskin with a relatively tight opening is pulled back and becomes trapped around the base of the glans. Once the glans begins to swell, this condition, called 'paraphimosis,' can rapidly become extremely painful; it requires medical advice as soon as possible.

Balanoposthitis is effectively treated with antibiotics by mouth. Paraphimosis requires a doctor to perform a special manoeuvre to get the foreskin back over the glans, perhaps with sedation or pain medication. For all these conditions, hygiene and comfort are best achieved by frequent, tepid, plain-water baths, and urination should be encouraged with the child sitting in the bath if urination is still painful.

Boys who have been circumcised may also have problems with painful urination. Occasionally they develop irritation and bleeding around the tip of the penis, at the opening of thc urethra, called 'meatal ulceration.' This generally occurs in young boys who are still in nappies, or in boys who frequently wet their clothing. The irritation appears to be caused by contact with urine trapped in the nappy or clothing. Treatment with skin protectants such as petroleum jelly, and attention to maintaining hygiene and minimising moisture and urine exposure, may reduce the problem.

 ## Does circumcision avoid problems, or cause them?

Some medical problems, such as urinary-tract infections and adult cancer of the penis, may occur more frequently in uncircumcised males. In addition to this, problems such as balanoposthitis and paraphimosis occur only in uncircumcised boys. Also, circumcised adult males are thought to have less risk of developing sexually transmitted diseases, including AIDS. Because of these concerns some doctors recommend circumcision of boys at birth. However, it's not at all clear whether circumcision can be justified for health reasons. For example, cancer of the penis is an extraordinarily rare condition that occurs much later in adulthood. Urinary-tract infections may be more prevalent in uncircumcised boys, but they are still uncommon and easy to treat, and there is no proof at all that they put uncircumcised boys at any higher risk of kidney scarring or other health problems. Even though circumcision is a relatively simple procedure, with few complications, the pain and risk of those complications (excessive bleeding, infection, and poor healing with scarring) must be balanced against the limited potential benefit.

However, certain boys may benefit from circumcision or related surgery. Those who have had an episode of balanoposthitis or paraphimosis may get it again, and may therefore benefit from circumcision. Also, a very small number of boys may benefit because the foreskin opening is so tight (called 'phimosis') that urination is messy or difficult, or retraction can't be achieved in adolescence. The decision must take many factors into account: how constant the problem is, the number of times it has occurred, the severity of the problem, and so on.

Some parents have social or religious reasons for circumcising their boys. Complications from the procedure are rare enough, and mostly mild enough, that such reasons are usually considered an acceptable basis for circumcision. Still, the procedure is not trivial, and not without some pain, even for newborn infants. There is evidence that medications such as local anaesthetics can significantly reduce the pain, and many doctors regard these as a necessary component of good medical care.

The issue of female circumcision

There is currently no proof that circumcision does any significant long-lasting harm, psychologically or physically, to most males. Female circumcision, which involves cutting away parts of the vulva and often includes sewing the opening of the vagina closed, or nearly closed, is a totally different procedure. Female circumcision can cause significant complications and suffering, both following the circumcision and throughout life. Because of this – despite the fact that female circumcision is culturally important in some societies – many medical organisations have taken a strong stand against the procedure, considering it unethical, and a case of malpractice for a doctor to participate in performing it.

Does circumcision make hygiene easier?

Bathing and hygiene of boys, circumcised or not, is not necessarily complicated. Though the connection is not as common or as obvious as with girls, non-specific irritants such as soaps and the trapping of moisture, or poor hygiene with toiletting, may contribute to irritation of the glans. The same general approaches used with girls, such as loose clothing with adequate air circulation to ensure drying, may be of use with boys. At birth the foreskin cannot easily be pulled back over the glans. However, as boys age the foreskin gradually becomes more mobile, and by three years of age it can usually be pulled back. However, regularly pulling the foreskin back or cleaning under it while bathing the child serves no clear purpose for most boys, and may occasionally cause additional irritation and problems.

Sexually transmitted infections can occur in sexually active or abused boys. Boys with painful urination who have been sexually active require assessment by a doctor able to deal with the multiple issues involved. Finally, testicular pain and/or swelling may occasionally be experienced by boys, though these conditions rarely involve painful urination. Unless these are brief, mild conditions obviously caused by minor injury, they require prompt medical advice.

CHAPTER 9

Sleeping Patterns and Problems

● ●

At one time or another, almost every parent has to deal with a child who has trouble falling asleep, or staying asleep through the night. When these problems persist, parents begin to worry about the child's well-being. They may also become exhausted themselves, so that the whole family is affected.

We still don't know exactly why we need to sleep, but we do know that people deprived of sleep become cranky and don't think very clearly.

We divide sleep into two main types – REM (rapid eye movement) sleep, during which we dream, and non-REM sleep, which makes us rested. Non-REM sleep varies from very light to very deep. During the night we go through repeated cycles of sleep, from light non-REM into deeper and deeper non-REM, and then into REM sleep and dreams. Between these cycles, we sometimes have brief periods of being awake.

A baby's cycle through the stages of non-REM sleep and then REM sleep and possible awakening generally takes 50 to 60 minutes. By adulthood this cycle lengthens to some 90 minutes. Babies spend about half their sleep time dreaming, but this declines as they get older; adolescents – like adults – dream for about 20 percent of their sleep time.

Children differ widely in the amount of sleep they need. The average baby sleeps about 16 hours out of 24, a one-year-old about 14 hours, a three-year-old about 12 hours. Under six months of age most children have three or four daytime naps a day, from 6 to 12 months they have about two naps, and sometime between three and four years of age they drop the daytime nap completely.

If you are hoping to change your child's sleep pattern, begin keeping a sleep diary to record the present pattern and any changes that develop. This

 84

way, you'll know if you're making progress. You'll find a sample sleep diary at the end of this chapter.

Why is it so hard to get some children to go to sleep?

If you have a toddler, you've probably faced endless bedtime requests for a drink of water, a trip to the bathroom, and so on. Difficulty in getting a child settled at night is a very common problem. Fortunately, it can usually be resolved with a structured bedtime routine.

The routine should last 15 to 20 minutes, and should be the same every night. For example, the child goes to the bathroom, completes tooth-brushing and face-washing, and gets into bed for a bedtime story; at the end of the story you turn out the light, give the child a good-night hug and kiss, and leave. A structured routine like this is very reassuring to a child, and means that both you and the child know what is expected and allowed.

But what if my child won't go to sleep in bed alone?

Once your child develops the habit of falling asleep under certain circumstances – such as in your arms, or in front of the television – you'll have to work to gradually modify that pattern and create the structured routine you want (see the discussion of maladaptive sleep associations, below).

What about a child who keeps waking up during the night?

Several studies have shown that it's common for children to wake up at night, especially between the ages of one and four; 10 percent of this age group awaken at least twice a night, and 30 percent at least three times a week. But the problem is not the fact that the child awakens – awakening between sleep cycles is normal, as noted earlier – but that he or she doesn't go back to sleep. These 'night awakenings' are the most common sleep disorder in children.

Unfortunately, night awakenings can be very persistent, and they often don't go away on their own; one study showed that 4 out of 10 children who had a problem with night awakenings at age eight months still had it at three years. The awakenings have been associated with several factors: difficulties at birth, developmental problems, parental depression, family stress, and the child having a difficult temperament.

Your response to a night awakening can also be an important factor. If you 'reward' the child – with a feeding, for example, or by bringing him or her back to your own bed, or by any other soothing contact – you're sending the child a message that waking up at night brings comfort and companion-ship. This is positive reinforcement of the waking-up habit.

Another factor in night awakenings is sleep associations – the bedtime conditions that the child typically falls asleep with. If these are conditions that he or she can't recreate alone, the normal awakenings that can come several times a night become traps that the child can't escape. Examples of such 'maladaptive' sleep associations include:

- being rocked in your arms;

- breast-feeding or bottle-feeding;

- being in another room or someone else's bed;

- using a dummy or pacifier the child can't replace;

- listening to music the child can't restart.

Often, positive reinforcement and maladaptive sleep associations com-bine to keep a child waking up. For example, a little boy falls asleep with a pacifier or dummy that rolls out of reach. When he has a normal night-time awakening, he can't get back to sleep without the dummy; he starts to fuss, and in comes a parent to retrieve the dummy and soothe him with back rubs and a lullaby. Is it any wonder he keeps waking up?

Preventing night awakenings

The key to preventing night awakenings is teaching your child to fall asleep alone at an early age. Even a baby 10 or 12 weeks old can be put into a cot or bassinette awake. To avoid creating positive reinforcement for waking,

- keep night-time encounters short and boring

- don't do unnecessary nappy changes at night

- try to drop night-time feedings after six months of age

- follow a consistent bedtime routine at the same time every evening

Q What can I do if my child already has poor sleep habits?

Several studies have shown that behaviour management is quite effective in treating frequent night awakenings. The basic principles are:

 86

1. identify the maladaptive sleep associations, and teach the child to fall asleep alone in circumstances he or she can re-create later in the night;

2. identify and gradually remove any positive reinforcement ('reward') for night awakenings.

In one study, parents of four-month-olds were encouraged to start putting their babies to bed partially awake so that they could learn to fall asleep by themselves; at nine months of age the babies were sleeping significantly better than a control group whose parents had not received such advice. In another study, the principles of teaching the child to sleep alone and removing positive reinforcers were applied to 19 children under the age of five who had a history of frequent night awakenings; researchers reported an 84 percent success rate, which was still maintained six months after the study ended.

Does that mean I should just leave the baby crying?

Letting a child 'cry it out' makes sense in terms of behaviour modification, as it removes the positive reinforcement of parental soothing and also leaves the child to get back to sleep without any maladaptive associations (food, dummy, etc.). One study divided children with night awakenings into two groups; the parents of Group One were told to leave their children crying, and the parents of Group Two were simply put on a waiting-list for treatment. The number of night awakenings in Group One decreased by 50 percent in the first week, and by 75 percent in the second week. However, some of the parents withdrew from the study when they learned that this was one of the treatments. In short, letting your baby 'cry it out' often works, but not all parents can bear to do it.

Are there more gradual ways to change my child's behaviour?

You can take things one at a time. Start by writing down your own analysis of the sleep problem: both the maladaptive sleep associations and the positive reinforcers. (For an example, see the box 'Changing Johnny's sleep habits.') This will give you a clear idea of what you need to change. Then tackle one new item every week or two.

It's essential that parents work together on this; it's difficult to deal with a screaming child *and* a screaming adult in the middle of the night!

Changing Johnny's sleep habits

Johnny is 14 months old. At nine months he started waking regularly at night, and now he's up three times a night. He goes to sleep well at bedtime; his parents hold him in their arms and give him a bottle, and move him to his cot once he's asleep. When he wakes up at night, they find that if they give him a bottle of formula he'll go back to sleep in five or 10 minutes; he generally finishes two eight-ounce bottles a night. Because they're exhausted by this regimen, his parents have recently started bringing him into bed with them.

Analysis of sleep problem

Maladaptive associations

● falling asleep on bottle

● falling asleep outside his cot

Positive reinforcers

● night-time feeding

● moving to parents' bed

Once Johnny's parents have analysed the problem, they can start changing their son's habits. First they gradually decrease his night-time feedings; then, step by step, they move him towards falling asleep in his own bed with no bottle, and staying there.

 How do I go about cutting out night-time feedings?

Healthy children over the age of six months don't need food at night. If this is one of the things you have to change, do it first; it's hard to make other behavioural changes when your child is looking for food. Make changes gradually, over one or two weeks.

If your child is on bottles, decrease the contents of each bottle by 20-30 mls each night; for example, two 150 ml bottles on Monday, two 120 ml bottles Tuesday, and so on, until you reach zero. This method is easier than watering down the formula, which leaves you with a child expecting water every night.

If your child is breast-fed, decrease the feeding time by one or two minutes a night; you can also lengthen the time between feeds by half an hour per night. Again, don't try to change other sleep habits until you've finished changing the feeding habits.

How do I get my child to fall asleep alone, if I can't bear to ignore the crying?

You can retrain your child by simply waiting a little longer each day before going in. This works best in a child under two who is still sleeping in a cot. (Don't use this method if your child is old enough to fall out of the cot.) Go through your normal bedtime routine and then put the child in the cot awake. Leave the room, but come back from time to time to reassure the child until he or she falls asleep – but stay only a minute or two each time, and don't pick the child up. Each visit should be brief but boring. Wait a little longer after each visit, and increase the intervals from night to night. For example:

	1st wait	*2nd wait*	*3rd wait*	*further waits*
Day 1	2 min.	4 min.	6 min.	6 min.
Day 2	4 min.	6 min.	8 min.	8 min.
Day 3	6 min.	8 min.	10 min.	10 min.
Day 4	8 min.	10 min.	12 min.	12 min.

Most children are quite upset during the first few nights of this change, but soon learn to fall asleep alone. The same technique can be used to decrease your response when the child wakes up during the night.

 ## But what if my child is already sleeping in a bed?

If you try the above method with an older child, he or she may follow you when you leave the room. Instead, you can try 'chair sitting.' Begin by sitting in a chair close to the child's bed – don't talk, just be there – and move the chair a foot farther away each night, until you're out of the room and down the hall. Children are rarely upset by this, as the change is so gradual. If a child does get up and follow you, give a warning the first time; after that, you can go out and hold the door closed for one minute and then return. If the child continues to follow you, increase the time you hold the door shut, until he or she stays quietly in bed.

Before you start this routine, explain the plan to the child; you may want to mark the final destination of your chair on the floor with masking tape. If the child is over three years old, it may help to offer a sticker as a reward for each night of co-operation.

If I cut out daytime naps, is my child more likely to sleep through the night?

Daytime naps generally shouldn't be more than two or three hours. Review your sleep diary. If your child is napping too much, gradually reducing nap time by five or 10 minutes a day may increase night-time sleeping. As a rule, children should be up by 8:00 A.M., and afternoon naps for those over a year old should end by 4:00 P.M.

Can I give my child sleeping medications?

Sleeping medications should not generally be used for children with night awakenings. They're effective, but once you take the child off the medication the problem usually starts again. Changing the child's behaviour patterns provides a lasting 'cure' and doesn't have the potential side-effects of medication.

What do I do if my child has nightmares?

Children sleep lightly during REM (dream) sleep, and may wake up screaming from nightmares. Bad dreams are especially distressing to toddlers, who can't understand the difference between dreams and reality. A child who is old enough to talk may be able to describe parts of the dream to you, so you can discuss it. In any case, your presence and reassurance will be comforting.

Recurrent nightmares are usually a sign that something is bothering the child; it may be minor, or something significant. With an older child, you can try talking about likely issues during the daytime, to relieve the stress. If the problem seems serious, consult your doctor.

What if the child is screaming in terror but doesn't seem awake?

Imagine that your child has been asleep for a couple of hours when you hear a blood-curdling scream. You rush to the bedroom and find the child sitting up, dripping with sweat, heart pounding. If the eyes are open, they look glazed and the pupils are dilated. Yet when you talk to the child you get no response. This is not a nightmare; it's a night terror.

Night terrors – which are classified as 'disorders of arousal' – happen when a child is in *non-dream* sleep, moving from a deeper stage to a lighter stage. No one really knows what causes them, but they're common in children aged 3 to 6 and gradually decrease after that. Though the child may be sitting up and wide-eyed, he or she is *not awake*, and is not aware of the surroundings. The episode may last as long as 20 or 30 minutes before the child falls back into 'peaceful' sleep. He or she will have no recollection of the terror the next morning.

Night terrors tend to come in clumps; there may be one or two a week for three or four months, and then they may disappear. There may be another series sometime later. A study of children who had recurring night terrors before the age of 10 found that, on average, they continued for 3.9 years. It also found that the children were emotionally normal. Night terrors tend to run in families.

What can I do about a night terror?

The first rule is to remain calm. Night terrors are very upsetting for parents, but remember: the child is asleep and will not remember this in the morning. Satisfy yourself that this is in fact a night terror; if the child is awake, the event was probably a nightmare. Night terrors can be confused with nighttime seizures, but children with seizures also have them in the daytime, and seizures often include urinating.

If it's a true night terror, stay in the room until it's over, and move breakables out of the way, but don't try to waken the child as this may prolong the episode. No further treatment is usually necessary, but if the episodes seem atypical, or a cycle lasts more than four months, you may want to consult your doctor.

Why do some children walk and talk in their sleep?

Like night terrors, sleepwalking and sleeptalking are disorders of arousal, and occur as the child moves from deep non-REM sleep to a lighter stage. The child usually wanders aimlessly and talks incoherently, and doesn't remember the episode the next day.

Because the child is asleep, he or she is unaware of danger, so it's up to you to take precautions. Supervise the child until he or she goes back to sleep, but don't try to wake the child up, as this may cause agitation. If you know a child sleepwalks, be sure doors and windows are securely locked, and take measures against any other hazards.

Most sleepwalkers are 10 to 12 years of age; sometimes sleepwalking begins as night terrors come to an end. There's usually a history of sleepwalking in the family. The condition doesn't seem to be linked to any emotional disorders, and no medical treatment is required.

Why do some babies rock and bang their heads when they're sleepy?

Rocking and head-banging are very common in young children, particularly boys; the behaviour tends to start after six months of age and disappears a few months later, but it sometimes goes on until the child is four or five.

Children usually rock by swinging back and forth in a crawling position. Those who bang their heads may also be in that position, or may be sitting up. Both behaviours are most common at bedtime, when the child is drowsy, but may also occur during the day or during a night awakening.

We don't know why some children bang their heads, but the actions may reflect the fact that rhythmic movements are soothing. The banging doesn't injure the child, although it may be hard on the walls and furniture. Almost all young head-bangers are emotionally well and developing normally. Although head-banging is more frequent in children with neurological problems such as autism and mental retardation, such conditions are usually obvious from daytime behaviour. There have been isolated cases of older head-bangers with emotional difficulties, but no good studies have been done.

There are no reported studies on treatment of head-banging. Most paediatricians recommend ignoring the behaviour, since it does no harm and eventually goes away; in any case, it's very hard to stop the child from doing it. If your child continues head-banging past the age of five, you should see your doctor, who can review the child's health and emotional status, and look for any stresses or anxieties.

When to see your doctor about sleep disorders

Sleep disorders are common in children, and most go away without treatment, but a few situations call for medical advice:

- persistent snoring or mouth-breathing
- night terrors lasting over four months
- persistent nightmares
- head-banging past five years of age
- concern about the child's emotional or general development

Sleep Diary

Please keep a record of your child's sleep patterns both day and night.

✗ – child put to bed

✓ – asleep

	Night					A.M.						Morning						P.M.					
	8	9	10	11	12	1	2	3	4	5	6	7	8	9	10	11	12	1	2	3	4	5	6	7
Week # ____																								
Sunday																								
Monday																								
Tuesday																								
Wednesday																								
Thursday																								
Friday																								
Saturday																								
Week # ____																								
Sunday																								
Monday																								
Tuesday																								
Wednesday																								
Thursday																								
Friday																								
Saturday																								
Week # ____																								
Sunday																								
Monday																								
Tuesday																								
Wednesday																								
Thursday																								
Friday																								
Saturday																								

CHAPTER 10

Skin: Spots and Rashes

kin problems are relatively common in children, and are often the cause of much parental concern. However, the vast majority are not serious. Many rashes don't bother the infant or child in the least, and most will disappear with no treatment. But some rashes are associated with serious diseases, and call for medical attention.

Q **What spots and rashes do newborns get?**

Chapter 2 described milia (like white or yellow pimples) and erythema toxicum (like red-rimmed pimples), which normally disappear soon after birth.

Mongolian spots are dark, pigmented patches of skin, usually on the lower back, buttocks, and legs. They are very common in Indian and Asian children but may occur in any race. They tend to fade with age. No complications are associated with them, and no treatment is necessary.

Vasomotor instability is often found in newborns and young infants. In this condition, the baby's skin may turn deep purple or red during crying; the hands and feet frequently look bluish, and the skin may be mottled. If the infant is otherwise well and vigorous, this is not a cause for concern.

Haemangiomas are abnormal collections of blood vessels that take several forms. The most common are 'salmon patches,' flat, pale pink 'birthmarks' on the back of the neck (sometimes called 'stork bites'), eyelids, forehead ('angel's kiss'), and nose. Those on the face usually fade and disappear by age two or three; those on the neck may not, but since they are usually covered by hair they are not unsightly.

'Port-wine stains' are flat, pink or reddish purple lesions, usually on the face. Since they don't fade, they may be a significant cosmetic problem. Laser

 94

therapy has recently been shown to be a safe and effective treatment for many port-wine stains.

'Strawberry' (capillary) haemangiomas are not usually present at birth, but appear within the first few weeks of life and may grow for several months. They are raised red or purplish marks that can occur anywhere on the face, body, or limbs. More than 90 percent will shrink and disappear partially or completely without leaving scars, so treatment is usually not indicated, but patience is very important. Medical intervention is sometimes necessary – if, for example, the haemangioma interferes with vision or breathing. Very rarely, these haemangiomas bleed or become infected.

 ### What other skin problems do small babies get?

Seborrhoeic dermatitis looks like yellow greasy scales, sometimes crusted. When it occurs on the scalp, it's known as 'cradle cap.' This rash may also occur in the creases of the nappy area and neck, and under the arms, and occasionally it affects the face. In these areas the rash often has a red, inflamed appearance, but it's not itchy or painful. Seborrhoeic dermatitis usually starts around four weeks of age, and has usually cleared up by one year.

Treatment is with moisturising creams or ointments. If the 'cradle cap' is very bad and shows no improvement, tar or salicylic acid–based shampoos may occasionally be applied (these should be used sparingly and carefully in infants). Keep in mind that seborrhoeic dermatitis bothers you much more than it bothers your baby! Other skin areas usually respond to steroid creams, which should be applied under the direction of a doctor.

A word about steroids

Steroids are cortisone-like medications that are often prescribed for skin problems. They are quite different from the steroids (androgens) that are used illegally by people trying to improve their strength or sporting abilities. Steroids used for medical purposes are available as skin creams, and as tablets or liquids to be taken by mouth. (Intravenous and inhaled steroids are also available, but these are seldom used for skin problems.) When prescribed and used appropriately, steroids are both safe and effective.

Nappy rashes include several different rashes that occur in the area covered by nappies. The rashes most frequently seen are 'nappy dermatitis' and 'candida dermatitis.'

'Nappy dermatitis' is probably due to pressure and irritation in the nappy region. It starts as shiny, reddish spots that may spread, join together, and become raw and painful. The skin creases are not usually involved. Nappy dermatitis usually appears in infants age 3 to 12 months, and prevention is easier than cure. The following measures may be helpful:

• Change nappies as frequently as possible (and reasonable), especially if the baby already has a rash or diarrhoea, or if you are using cloth nappies.

• Avoid tight-fitting nappies.

• Avoid irritating soaps; wash the skin with warm water only.

• Try to keep the skin dry.

Barrier creams containing zinc oxide are most useful after a rash has set in. Once the baby is out of nappies, this rash will not recur.

'Candida dermatitis' (thrush) is due to a yeast, which thrives in warm moist environments such as the nappy area. It can also occur in other areas, including the mouth. In the nappy area, it starts in the creases and spreads outward. Little pimples or pustules are often seen at the edges; the rash itself is often red and raw. Some babies develop candida nappy rashes after taking oral antibiotics.

Treatment is with antifungal creams. Some doctors recommend using a steroid cream in combination with an antifungal agent, but no studies have been done to determine which is the best method of treatment. Oral medications are not necessary unless there is evidence of thrush in the baby's mouth.

Babies with frequently recurring candida infections, or infections that don't clear up with treatment, should be seen by a doctor.

 Why do some babies have patches of different skin colour?

Normal skin colour is mainly due to a pigment called 'melanin.' Uneven skin colour can result from too much or too little pigment in small or large areas of the body. These may be present at birth or develop later. In some people, injuries heal with areas of increased or decreased pigment. Aside from the cosmetic aspect, most abnormalities of pigment are not a cause for concern. Sometimes, though, they are associated with underlying illnesses, or increased risk of certain diseases. For this reason, it's a good idea to point out areas of different skin colour to your doctor.

Why do some babies have a lot of body hair?

The vast majority of children who appear 'hairy' are quite normal. Frequently, other members of their family are hairy too. There is a large variation in the amount of body hair between different racial and ethnic groups. Western society, unfortunately, favours less body hair, particularly in women – hence the large market for hair-removing products.

Occasionally, diseases cause excess body hair. In some cases the illness is obvious (for example, severe malnutrition or anorexia nervosa can result in increased hairiness). Also, some medications cause increased body hair. If the increased hair growth is all over the body, it is called 'hypertrichosis.' If it's in the genital area, under the arms, or on the face, it is called 'hirsutism.'

You should be concerned about your child having too much body hair only if there is any indication the child may be ill, or if hirsutism occurs in a child who is too young to be entering puberty.

Aren't some rashes caused by allergies?

Atopic dermatitis (eczema) is by definition an extremely itchy skin rash. It can occur in all age groups, but is more common in infants and young children and usually starts within the first year of life. The site and appearance of the rash vary with age: in infants the face is most often involved; in older children the crooks of the elbows and backs of the knees are typically affected. In young children the rash often looks moist, whereas in older ones the skin appears hard and thickened. Scratching may cause the rash to become infected. Itching is often provoked by changes in temperature, fabrics like wool, and some soaps. Although the cause of atopic dermatitis is unknown, it is frequently associated with asthma and allergies.

Atopic dermatitis tends to improve with age, although in a large number of affected children it persists into or recurs in adulthood. The most important part of treatment is preventing itching. Try to keep the child in cotton clothes, and apply moisturising creams generously to the child's body after bathing. Have the bath water tepid – hot water will increase the irritation. Pat the dry skin gently after bathing and apply the emollient cream within three minutes of getting out of the bath. Some creams will cause the child to itch more and may burn or inflame the skin. If any irritation occurs, discontinue using it and try an alternative brand. Many pharmacies have sample sizes of products that you can try. Corticosteroids are the mainstay of treatment – lotions, creams, ointments, and gels are available in varying strengths – but these should be used sparingly for as short a time as possible, as long-term use may damage the skin or have other side-effects. Antihistamines may be used, especially at night; they don't appear to have a direct effect on the skin disease but do improve sleep. To reduce scratching, keep the child's nails short. Some parents find it helpful to put mittens on the hands of small children at night.

Approximately 60 percent of children under the age of five with *severe* eczema have an underlying food allergy. It may help to see a specialist to identify whether food is a likely cause and whether it is necessary to modify the child's diet. This should be done in consultation with a registered dietitian.

Contact dermatitis is an allergic skin reaction to a particular substance. Common causes include poison ivy, nickel (in jewellery, zippers, or fasteners), and cosmetics. The rash usually appears at a site that has been directly exposed, although similar rashes sometimes develop in unexposed areas of skin. The affected skin is red and swollen, and blisters may form. It's extremely itchy. Allergic contact dermatitis is unusual in children under the age of five.

Treatment is by avoiding the allergen, or removing it and thoroughly washing the affected area. Cool compresses and steroid creams may be used to relieve the symptoms. In severe cases (such as a bad case of poison ivy), a doctor can prescribe further treatment.

Urticaria (hives) is another allergic response that may be due to a number of causes, including food, drugs, insect bites, and viral infections. In contrast to contact dermatitis, direct skin contact is not necessary to produce this rash; for example, some people get hives after taking an antibiotic like penicillin by mouth. The rash consists of raised pink spots with pale centres (weals), which may be quite small or very large. The rash may come and go, and the size, shape, and site of the lesions can change very rapidly. It's very itchy, and usually lasts for two or three days.

In some children the cause of hives is obvious, but in many cases the allergic agent is never found. Many children develop hives only once. Antihistamines such as Benadryl are helpful for hives, but if the cause is known, avoiding it obviously makes more sense. An allergy specialist can do tests to identify the cause of the reaction.

Occasionally, hives form part of a potentially life-threatening allergic reaction. If the child appears sick or has any difficulty breathing, or has swelling of the lips or tongue, medical help should be sought urgently. You should also consult a doctor if the reaction appears to be due to a medication, or if there are accompanying symptoms such as joint swelling and fever.

What else causes an itchy red rash?

Scabies is another cause. The rash is extremely itchy, especially at night, and looks like small, reddish, raised bumps. It's caused by tiny mites (bugs) that burrow into the skin. In older children, scabies most commonly occurs between the fingers, on the inner surface of the wrists, and in the armpits, abdomen, groin, and buttocks. In children younger than two, the rash may look like little blisters, and is likely to occur on the head and neck, palms, and soles. The infection is transmitted from person to person by close contact.

The treatment of choice is permethrin cream, which appears to be the safest drug available for the purpose. The cream should be applied to the entire body below the head for children older than two years; the entire head and neck should be included for younger children. The cream should be washed off by bathing after 8 to 14 hours. It's important to follow the instructions closely. It is recommended that *all* household members be treated at the same time, and all bedding and clothing should be washed and dried at hot temperatures, to kill any remaining mites.

 ## What if my child has a rash and a fever?

Rash and fever are prominent features of many childhood infections. The vast majority are caused by viruses. It's often possible to distinguish these illnesses by differences in the rashes, and associated features such as joint pain and conjunctivitis (red, irritated eyes, with or without mucus). However, it's sometimes difficult to make a specific diagnosis, because many viruses produce similar types of diseases. The descriptions below will give you an idea of what disease your child may have; for information on the seriousness, side-effects, and treatment of these diseases, see Chapter 14, 'Diseases and Medical Conditions.'

A low fever soon accompanied by a rash of *raised red bumps that become little fluid-filled blisters* suggests chickenpox. The rash usually starts on the trunk and face, and then spreads to the rest of the body.

***

Meningococcal disease in New Zealand

Any child with a fever and a purple or red rash should be seen immediately by a doctor or emergency clinic. This could be a sign of meningococcal sepsis or meningitis. There is an epidemic of this life threatening infection in New Zealand at present (February 2000).

How can I tell if a rash is serious?

It's important to look at the 'company a rash keeps.' If a child is well, happy, and active, you needn't worry unduly about a spot or rash that he or she hasn't even noticed! There are times, however, when you should be concerned about a rash.

Seek medical help immediately if a child also has any of the following:

- a change in level of consciousness
- extreme irritability or sleepiness
- swelling of the lips or tongue
- difficulty breathing
- bleeding or bruising
- severe headache or neck pain

Seek medical help soon if a child also has any of the following:

- sores on the lips or in the mouth, eyes, or genital area
- blistering or peeling of the skin
- joint pain and/or swelling
- blood in the urine
- fever that doesn't go away within a couple of days
- pain
- ongoing vomiting and/or diarrhoea
- a known immune disorder

Seek medical help before too long if any of the following occurs:

- a skin rash doesn't go away, or keeps coming back
- a mole or spot gets bigger, changes colour, or bleeds
- a child has areas of increased or decreased pigmentation
- the child is not growing well
- you are concerned about the cosmetic appearance of a spot or rash

A fine pink or red rash that begins on the face and feels like sandpaper, accompanied by fever, headache, vomiting, and sore throat, likely indicates scarlet fever. A few days later, the tongue becomes red and swollen.

Fine, pale pink spots on the face and hairline, which later spread to the rest of the body and may join up into solid pink patches, suggest rubella (German measles). There may or may not be fever.

A reddish rash that spreads down from the scalp, hairline, and neck, preceded by high fever, runny nose, cough, and red eyes, probably means the child has measles. A few days later, small white spots appear in the mouth.

A bright red rash on the face, mainly the cheeks, preceded by low fever and a sore throat, suggests fifth disease. A lacy rash may appear on the limbs and trunk.

A fine pink or reddish rash that spreads from the trunk to the neck and

limbs, preceded by a high fever, may mean roseola; the disease is rare in children over the age of four.

What can I do if my child has sunburn?

The severity of sunburn ranges from mild redness of the skin, to redness with pain and swelling and sometimes blistering. If a large area of skin has been burned, the child may feel ill and have a headache, nausea, fever, and chills. The effects are usually seen 6 to 12 hours after overexposure to the sun, and may get worse over the next few days. Peeling of the skin frequently follows.

Treatment is aimed at keeping the child as comfortable as possible until the skin heals. Cool baths or wet compresses may be helpful. Non-prescription (0.5 percent) steroid creams may decrease the redness and swelling. Anti-inflammatory drugs such as ASA and ibuprofen may be useful, but you should discuss them with your doctor (see the note on ASA in Chapter 5). Paracetamol can be given to provide some pain relief.

Prevention is really the key. In addition to causing painful burns, sunburn can contribute to several types of skin cancer later in life. Children under the age of six months should be kept out of the sun as much as possible; sunscreens are not recommended for this age group. For older children, current recommendations say that sunscreens with a sun protection factor (SPF) of over 15 should be applied to exposed areas 30 to 60 minutes before they go into the sun, and that the sunscreens should be reapplied every 60 to 90 minutes. After swimming or extensive perspiration, even 'waterproof' sunscreens should be reapplied.

What about unusually dry skin?

Skin dryness is due to loss of water from the outer layers of the skin. Some families have a tendency to dry skin and chapping. Environmental factors including heat, humidity, and soap also play an important role.

The areas most affected are usually the hands, arms, and shins, which may look as if they're covered by fine, flaky scales. Dry skin isn't usually irritating, although it sometimes itches. If the problem is severe, the skin may actually crack, creating painful sores.

As with sunburn, prevention is easier than cure. You can keep room temperatures as low as comfortably possible, since heat has a drying effect, and you may find humidifiers useful. (Remember to clean your humidifier regularly, as it can be a source of mould.) Children with dry skin should not be bathed more than once every two days. Try to avoid excessive exposure to soaps. (There is no scientific evidence that one soap is better than another, for normal children.) Bath oils can be added to the water, but remember that they make the bathtub slippery and dangerous. Moisturising lotions or creams should be applied to the child's skin after bathing, while the skin is still moist.

It is important to identify whether the dry skin may, in fact, be eczema, which can sometimes present itself as very dry skin. A good emollient cream should then be applied generously within three minutes of getting out of the bath.

If dry skin doesn't improve after a few weeks of the above measures, contact your doctor. Some authorities recommend moving to a subtropical climate, especially during the winter. Unfortunately, this isn't a practical option for most of us!

 ## Is there any remedy for acne?

Acne is probably the most common skin disorder, occurring in more than 85 percent of teenagers. Although girls are affected at a younger age than boys, severe acne is more common in boys. The cause of acne is not well understood, but it's probably due to a combination of hormonal changes and infection. Acne also occurs in young babies, probably due to the mothers' hormones. There is no evidence to support the popular belief that acne is caused by certain foods (such as chocolate) or by dirt.

Several types of spots occur in acne, including blackheads, whiteheads, pimples, and cysts. Acne can be itchy or painful, and a severe case may result in scarring. The face is most commonly affected; the back, neck, chest, and shoulders may also be involved.

Treatment of acne depends on its severity, and on how concerned the patient is. Some people find that exposure to the sun improves their acne; humidity and greasy ointments may be aggravating. Certain medications (most commonly hormones) can cause or worsen acne.

Benzoyl peroxide and antibiotic creams have been shown to be useful in treating acne. Exfoliating agents like tretinoin and salicylic acid, which cause irritation of the skin followed by peeling, are also used. For more severe forms of acne, adding oral antibiotics may be helpful. Isotretinoin (Accutane) is effective for very severe acne, but it can cause major birth defects if taken during pregnancy; therefore teens should be warned *never* to share their medication.

Babies with acne don't require any treatment, since the spots will disappear on their own. Acne in teenagers usually improves by the late teens or early twenties.

CHAPTER 11

Problems with Eyes and Ears

●●●●●●●●●●●●●●●●●●●●●●●●●●●●●●●

Children's eyes and ears deserve special attention, not only because they are delicate and easily damaged, but also because the input they provide is essential to a child's development. Since babies can't tell us if they are seeing or hearing poorly, it's up to parents to watch for signs that their children aren't responding normally to sights and sounds.

Eye Problems
●●●●●●●●●●●●●●●●●●●

A child's eye problems sometimes begin at birth, when an eye infection may be picked up during passage through the birth canal. Such infections can be very serious, although they respond well to treatment. If your baby has a yellowish discharge from the eyes, notify your doctor.

Q **What if one of my baby's eyes is always watering?**

Excessive tearing is a very common problem in the first year of life, and is usually limited to one eye. Tears are normally secreted to keep the eye clean and moist, and drain from the eyes into the nose. In some babies, however, the tear-duct system fails to open completely, so that tears accumulate in the eyes. Your doctor can show you how to massage the lacrimal sac and tear-duct system so the tears drain as they should.

Sometimes the eyes have a coloured discharge as well, which may require a prescription of antibiotic drops. In most cases, massage and antibiotic drops will solve the problem. If persistent tearing continues until the child is 12 to 15 months old, a relatively simple procedure of probing the tear duct can be carried out by an eye doctor.

103

When do babies start to see?

Babies can see at birth, though they don't have normal adult vision. Newborns can see large shapes – particularly faces, which have strong visual appeal. They appreciate strong, bright colours more readily than lighter shades. Visual development occurs very rapidly during the first year of life; by three months of age an infant will follow objects such as a ball or mobile in his or her line of vision. If your baby doesn't track objects in the visual field by this age, bring this to the doctor's attention.

 What does it mean if my child's eyes are red?

A red or 'bloodshot' eye is common, but should be checked by the doctor. Red eyes associated with tearing and itching, and particularly nasal congestion, indicate an allergic problem – often hay fever, asthma, or eczema. Treatment may include oral antihistamine-like medications or eye drops, or a combination of both.

A red or bloodshot eye may also be due to an infection, often contracted through contact with another child in the family or at the daycare centre. Careful hand-washing is essential in treating these infections, as they are easily spread to the rest of the family.

Bacterial eye infections are usually associated with a discharge that is thick and yellow in colour, and crusts the eyelid margins, particularly on awakening in the morning. This sort of infection is often accompanied by an upper-respiratory-tract infection. Treatment consists of bathing the eye in warm water, and sometimes oral antibiotics as well as antibiotic eye drops. Any child who has red eyes and significant yellow eye discharge should be assessed by a doctor.

Often a viral infection causes conjunctivitis with a prominent discharge, usually watery. Local lymph nodes may be swollen. Again the condition is highly infectious, and may spread through families and daycare centres. These viral infections are usually self-limiting, and no specific treatment is indicated.

Whether the infection is thought to be bacterial or viral, a child with discharge from the eye should be kept away from other children to avoid spreading the condition.

A red eye can also be caused by inflammation of the eyelid (blepharitis), a condition involving the eyelashes and surrounding glands. This is often associated with a scaling skin condition such as seborrhoea, or with a chronic bacterial infection of the eyelids. As the condition progresses there may be crusting and discharge, and the child may complain of itching in the eye. This type of infection is treated with local antibiotics.

Scaling skin around the eyes – often a greasy, dandruff-like scale on the lashes – may be associated with scaling of the scalp and ears. It's best treated by scrubbing the lid margins nightly for a month with a cotton swab and a non-irritating baby shampoo.

What if there's a boil on the eyelid?

This is a sty, a localised infection of the eyelid that also involves the surrounding glands. The whole eyelid is usually red, swollen, and tender. You can apply warm compresses for 15 minutes four times a day, and a local antibiotic may be prescribed. A sty generally drains within a few days. If it persists for several weeks, your doctor may refer you to an eye doctor.

Do red eyes ever indicate a serious problem?

More serious conditions are due to bacterial infection of the tissues surrounding the eye or eye socket. They are usually associated with a high fever; the child appears ill and there may be swelling or protrusion of the eye. The skin around the eye is red. These infections sometimes follow injury to the eye area, or a respiratory infection involving the sinuses, which are close to the eye. They must be assessed by a doctor immediately, and appropriate antibiotic therapy must be given, usually in hospital.

A persistent red eye that is not associated with a discharge may indicate a more complicated eye problem, particularly if there is pain and sensitivity to light, or decreased vision. This calls for immediate attention from an eye specialist.

Should I worry if my baby's eyes seem crossed?

During well-baby visits, the doctor will be checking to see that your baby's eyes are working together and that there is good sight in each eye. Though an infant's eyes may not be co-ordinated in the first few months of life, persistence of a 'crossed' eye after the age of six months should be brought to the doctor's attention, as should any family history of visual problems.

Crossed eyes (also called strabismus or squint) indicate that the eye muscles are not properly aligned, so that one eye deviates from its normal position. However, some children whose eyes appear crossed merely have a broad, flat nasal bridge, creating the illusion of crossed eyes. As the nose matures, this appearance goes away. Let the doctor decide whether your baby really has crossed eyes, or just a broad nasal ridge. If the eyes are crossed beyond six months of age, the condition will not go away without treatment by an eye doctor.

It's important to treat crossed eyes because the misalignment presents the brain with two different images. Since the brain has trouble processing these two images at the same time, it will gradually suppress the images from one eye, leading to a marked reduction in vision in that eye.

Crossed eyes can sometimes be corrected non-surgically, with eye patches and eyeglasses, but surgery may be required when non-surgical methods don't work.

 When should my child's vision first be checked?
In addition to the checks done at well-baby visits in the first two years of life, a child's vision may be evaluated by 3 to 4 years of age. For example, the child may be shown a large letter E in various positions and taught to point his or her fingers in the same direction as the 'fingers' of the E. This may require some advance practice with parents, so that the child feels ready to co-operate. Pictures are used as well, though this depends on the maturity of the child; some young patients don't co-operate because of lack of experience with the pictures, or an inability to name them.

 Can't I wait to see if visual problems go away on their own?
Your child's psychological and learning development requires normal, co-ordinated vision. If visual defects aren't corrected early, development may be seriously impaired. Worse yet, there may be permanent damage to your child's vision.

 Aren't there eye exercises to correct learning problems?
The use of exercises to compensate for specific learning and reading disabilities is not as yet supported by scientific evidence.

Ear Problems
. . . .
Ear infections (otitis media) are the bacterial infections that most often bring children to the doctor in the first three years of life. Most occur between the ages of six months and two years, and children who have their first attack before the age of one are more likely to have recurrent infections than those who have their first bout later.

The anatomy of the ear

The ear has three main areas – outer (the ear canal we can see), middle (where sounds are transmitted from the eardrum by a delicate arrangement of bones), and inner (where sound signals are passed to the auditory nerve and the brain). The middle ear is connected to the throat by the eustachian tube. If the outside pressure changes (when we go up in an aeroplane, for example), the difference between outer-ear pressure and inner-ear pressure pushes on the eardrum, making us uncomfortable. Older children learn to 'equalise' this pressure by yawning or swallowing to let air from the throat into the eustachian tubes; it's not so easy to manoeuvre infants into opening their eustachian tubes. Swelling or congestion of the eustachian tube can make equalisation impossible, so that pressure differences create pain.

Bones Conveying Sound

Auditory Nerve (Leading to Brain)

Eustachian Tube

External Ear

Eardrum

Middle Ear

Inner Ear

Outer Ear Canal

Why do young children have so many ear infections?

There are many contributing factors. Children in this age group have fairly low levels of protective antibodies, and increasing exposure to respiratory infections in daycare and other gatherings. Their eustachian tubes are relatively short and have less supporting cartilage; the cartilage keeps the tube open because it is fairly rigid. With less cartilage, it's like a kinked hose. Any upper-respiratory-tract infection causes congestion of the lining of the respiratory tract and eustachian tube, making fluid accumulate in the middle ear. Germs proliferate in these secretions, and ear infections are the result.

Other factors, such as respiratory allergies and underlying anatomical defects (a cleft palate, for example), sometimes account for recurrent ear infections. Secondary cigarette smoke and excess humidity may be factors as well. (Cigarette smoke affects the protective lining of the eustachian tube so that bacteria can't easily be removed by the cells of the lining.)

It's true that infants and young children have relatively more lymphoid tissue, such as adenoids and tonsils, to protect the respiratory tract and help in the production of antibodies. However, these tissues – particularly the adenoids, when they're swollen – can obstruct the eustachian tube and further block drainage.

 Does breast-feeding help prevent ear infections?

The role of breast-feeding in protecting against ear infections is somewhat controversial; so is the role of food allergies.

 When are ear infections most likely?

Most occur during the 'cold season,' because of the frequency of respiratory infections at that time of year. Most ear infections are initiated by viral infections or mild upper-respiratory-tract infections (colds). Usually there is a slight fever and some nasal congestion, and the youngster becomes increasingly irritable and unhappy, sleeping and feeding poorly, and often developing a higher temperature. The fact that an infant pulls on his or her ear is not a reliable sign of an ear infection, but an older child will give verbal or other indications of pain in the affected ear. He or she should be seen by a doctor, who will diagnose the ear infection by examining the child and observing the eardrum and its mobility.

It's sometimes very difficult to examine the eardrum of a young infant or child. Proper examination may be possible only after removing wax from the ear canal by careful syringing by the child's doctor.

Treatment will be a 10-day course of an appropriate antibiotic, with follow-up by the doctor in 2 to 6 weeks. The child's discomfort and fever can be treated with paracetamol. If the nose is badly blocked, a saline nose-drop preparation may help, or excess mucus may be aspirated (sucked out). There is increasing evidence that ear infections may resolve spontaneously without antibiotics, and some doctors will elect not to treat initially but review in 24 hours when antibiotics will be prescribed if there is ongoing evidence of otitis media. The child should show improvement within 48 hours. If there is persistent fever or a worsening of the symptoms after that time, the child must be reassessed to be certain that the prescribed medication is appropriate, and that no more serious complication has developed.

 Are these antibiotics safe?
Some parents are reluctant to have their child on antibiotics, particularly for recurrent bouts of ear infections over a relatively long period of time. Remember that your doctor is very aware of the possible side-effects of antibiotics; your child's medical history, particularly any previous allergy to a medication or any significant side-effect, will be taken into account. Antibiotic therapy can prevent chronic mastoid infection, draining ears, and major hearing loss. Even life-threatening complications of ear infections, such as brain abscess and meningitis, have decreased significantly because of antibiotics.

 What happens once my child is on antibiotics?
By the follow-up examination two weeks later, there is usually marked improvement, although some fluid may remain in the middle ear. If this is the case, the doctor will follow the child's progress over the next few months to be sure the fluid drains. If fluid is still present after three months, the child may need a hearing test to see whether the quantity of fluid is significant. If hearing is being affected, a long-term course of low-dose antibiotics may clear it up, avoiding the need for surgery.

 Can decongestants or antihistamines be used for middle-ear infections?
The use of oral decongestants and antihistamines for these infections has not been shown to be effective. In addition, many of these medications cause side-effects such as drowsiness, excitability, and irritability, which make the child's condition more difficult to evaluate.

What happens if my child keeps getting ear infections?

Children who have frequent bouts of ear infection, particularly over the winter months, may be given a course of prophylactic (preventive) antibiotics. This approach is particularly effective in children aged six months to four years who have more than three bouts in a six-month period. These antibiotics are safe and inexpensive; just half the usual dose is given, once a day.

Children who keep getting ear infections even with prophylactic antibiotics may need surgery to drain the ears and insert ventilating tubes (grommets) through the eardrum and into the middle ear. This is the commonest operation performed on children today, and is very safe, but it should be undertaken only after evaluation by the child's doctor in consultation with an ear, nose, and throat specialist. They will consider not only the number of ear infections, but hearing problems, the persistence of thick fluid in the middle ear, reduced mobility of the eardrum, and persistent abnormal or negative pressure in the middle ear.

If tubes are inserted, they usually fall out or are removed after a few months, and the holes in the eardrum heal naturally.

About 10 percent of children later require a further set (or sets) of ventilating tubes. In this case, another course of prophylactic antibiotics should be considered, particularly over the winter, when respiratory infections are common.

 Why all this fuss over an ear infection?

Children with ear infections are irritable and have a significant amount of pain. They need quick and efficient treatment to relieve their symptoms, and to keep the ear infection from leading to more serious problems. Also, an aggressive approach to the infection may keep the child from missing valuable time at school or daycare.

Some children with recurrent bouts of ear infection, and associated abnormalities of middle-ear pressure, exhibit behavioural changes. Whether their language and speech development suffers is less clear, although there is of course concern that significant hearing loss in both ears may account for some delay. There is as yet no agreement as to the minimum hearing sensitivity that infants and young children need for the complex process of developing speech and language successfully.

All children who have recurrent bouts of ear infection should be evaluated for middle-ear fluid. This can be done by observing the eardrum and evaluating middle-ear pressure by tympanometry (a technique using air pressure). Hearing evaluation by audiometry, using an electronic device that produces sounds for the child to hear, may also be necessary.

Are all ear infections in the middle ear?

Infections of the ear canal, commonly called 'swimmer's ear,' are often seen in the summer months. These can cause extreme pain, due to inflammation and the accumulation of debris in the ear canal. Treatment consists of painkillers, irrigation (flushing out) of the debris, and use of a combination ear drop containing antibiotics and cortisone.

What about other kinds of hearing problems?

Babies in high-risk groups – those with a family history of hearing loss or deafness, premature infants, and infants who need treatment in a neonatal intensive care unit – should be observed for possible hearing deficiency in the first few months of life.

Your own observations of your infant are very important in assessing his or her response to voices and general noise, and your intuitions are valuable. Any concerns you have about the baby's response to verbal or other stimulation should be brought to the attention of the doctor.

Most toddlers have a vocabulary of about 10 words by 18 months and twice as many words by 21 months. By two years of age, most are linking a couple of words together. If your child is slow to reach these milestones, point this out to the doctor. A complete evaluation will include an ear, nose, and throat examination and a full assessment of the child's social and psychological background.

Toddlers who show delay in language development should have their hearing assessed by audiometry. Note, however, that infants from disadvantaged social situations or chaotic home environments may be delayed in language development. Some children who are constantly exposed to another language, perhaps from babysitters or grandparents, show a delay in language development, but they usually catch up by the age of four or five.

CHAPTER 12

Feeding Your Child

O ne of the most exciting things about being a parent is watching your children develop. Children grow and change quite quickly; 'My, how you've grown!' is the stock exclamation of grandparents who don't see their grandchildren on a daily basis. Since newborns may weigh as little as 600 gm (1½ pounds), between birth and age 18 (when most children have completed their growth), a child's weight may multiply by 20 to 100 times. Genes inherited from parents determine many physical characteristics (height and weight, and colour of hair, eyes, and skin), but a major factor influencing children's growth is their nutrition.

Obviously children need the right nutrients for growth, and to provide energy for daily activities. But they also need to acquire good eating habits, which will have a strong impact on their future food choices and health. Feeding infants and young children also helps them feel secure that they are loved. Feeding should be a time of happiness and pleasure, a time to promote love and security; it is not a time for speed, efficiency, or neatness. Food should be enjoyed!

Q How do I get my child to eat the right foods?

Although you should make sure your child gets a complete and well-balanced diet, you needn't be overly anxious or particular about what he or she eats. Children have a natural tendency to eat the right foods, in suitable amounts. Despite cultural diversity and varied ethnic traditions around the world, most societies have come up with appropriate diets. What a child in New Zealand and a vegetarian child in south Asia eat may be very different, but each diet may be ideally suited for the child in question. But keep in mind the fact that children learn by example. If you want your children to develop healthy, nutritious eating habits, you have to set an example.

How do I know if I'm choosing the right foods?

Our food can be considered in terms of carbohydrates, proteins, fats, vitamins, and minerals. Carbohydrates, in simple sugar forms or in complex starch forms, provide energy. Proteins are used to build and repair the body. Fats are used as more concentrated sources of energy, and to build certain body structures, such as the brain and nervous tissue. Vitamins (A, the B group, C, D, E, and K) and minerals (sodium, potassium, iron, calcium, magnesium, and others) are used in the normal growth and maintenance of our bodies. As a general rule, you don't have to worry about exactly what your child eats, as long as his or her diet accords with the New Zealand guidelines for healthy infants, toddlers and children, which suggest a reasonable balance of breads, cereals, and grains for energy; protein foods like meat, fish, or beans for body growth; fruits and vegetables for vitamins and minerals; and milk and dairy products for all these benefits. Most New Zealand children who eat a balanced diet get adequate vitamins, so vitamin supplements are not usually required for healthy children.

Feeding an Infant

'Breast Is Best' is a slogan used by most paediatricians; all mothers should be encouraged to breast-feed. Breast milk is perfectly suited for the newborn, and – in spite of science and advertising – no other infant food is superior to human milk. It provides the ideal combination of essential proteins, fats, and carbohydrates for newborns, as well as some natural protection against infections. For the child with an inherited tendency to allergic reactions such as eczema or asthma, breast milk has fewer allergenic substances than cow's milk or soy-based formula (although there is little solid evidence that breast-feeding actually protects infants from such allergic conditions). Finally, breast-feeding encourages bonding between mother and child, helps mothers understand the cues infants give regarding their needs, and can be very convenient for both mother and infant. It's also inexpensive.

 Can babies breast-feed right from birth?

During the first week, breast-feeding may not be easy. Very little breast milk is produced in the first two days. Also, it may be difficult for a newborn to latch on to the mother's breast, and some mothers find it uncomfortable. It's important to get prenatal and postnatal teaching and help from the midwife, lactation consultant or plunket nurse during the first few weeks at home.

Do breast-feeding babies need extra vitamins and minerals?

Fluoride is important for developing teeth, and adding fluoride to the water supply in most communities has resulted in a lower rate of children's dental cavities. If your water supply is low in fluoride, a flouride supplement may be appropriate. Note that, as with most substances, too much can create a problem. Excess fluoride can cause tooth discolouring called 'fluorosis.' You should discuss the need for fluoride supplements with your doctor or dentist.

Breast milk has little iron, but the iron in it is much more readily absorbed than other forms of iron in food. For the first six months of life, there is enough iron in breast milk to allow for normal growth and normal production of red blood cells. However, some newborns – especially premature and low-birthweight infants – have only a small amount of iron stored in their bodies, and require iron supplements. By 4 to 6 months of age, most infants should be started on solid foods that contain iron. In New Zealand this usually means prepared infant cereals, which are fortified with iron. Rich sources of iron include lean lamb, beef and chicken.

 ### Are there reasons not to breast-feed?

Some women prefer not to breast-feed because of previous negative experience, personal feelings, breast surgery, etc. Others who are ill or have nipple abnormalities have difficulties breast-feeding. If you are taking medications on a regular basis, discuss this with your doctor; most medications, including alcohol and nicotine, pass into the breast milk. If you are on hormones, or drugs for cancer, thyroid disease, or certain psychiatric illnesses, you may be advised not to breast-feed.

 ### How long should babies breast-feed?

It is recommended that infants be exclusively breast fed from birth to 4 to 6 months of age and preferably up to 12 months of age. Appropriate weaning solids should be introduced around 4 to 6 months.

The New Zealand Plunket child health study found that although breast feeding rates were high at birth (98 percent were exclusively breast fed at birth) they declined significantly with time after birth. At six weeks, 69 percent were exclusively breast fed; 49 percent at three months. By six months 2.5 percent of infants were exclusively fed and 56 percent of infants were still receiving some breast milk.

Hints on breast-feeding

- Breast-milk production does not 'turn on' until the third or fourth day, but during this interval a small amount of fluid called 'colostrum,' high in energy and antibodies, is flowing. The newborn doesn't need a lot of fluid; there is an excess in the tissues at birth, which is why most babies lose up to 10 percent of their birthweight in the first two or three days of life.

- Not all babies learn immediately to 'latch on' to the breast. Some authorities feel that giving bottles, or even pacifiers or dummies, too early can cause further confusion.

- In the early days or weeks it's best to feed 'on demand' (but at least every four or five hours). With time, the frequency of feeding will naturally decrease from every two hours to every four. By six months of age, your baby will likely be sleeping 8 to 10 hours at night.

- When feeding or crying, babies may swallow lots of air. Most of it passes into the bowel and is absorbed. Some may remain in the stomach, taking up space and making your baby feel full. Burping after feeding from the first breast is helpful, but you should persist for only two or three minutes before carrying on with the feed.

- Unlimited suckling from the beginning has been shown to improve the success rate of breast-feeding, and does not lead to sore nipples. Sore nipples are usually from improper positioning of the infant on the breast. The baby should suck on the dark portion of the breast (the areola) behind the nipple.

- The baby will empty the breast in 6 to 8 minutes. The highest fat content of breast milk is in the last portion of the feeding. Try feeding the baby 10 minutes on one side, burping the baby, then nursing for 10 to 15 minutes on the other side.

- In the early stages there may be more milk than the baby needs. This may be a good time to pump the excess and store it in the freezer; it can be stored for up to six months. Do not thaw it in the microwave!

- A baby wets 6 to 8 nappies per day if he or she is getting enough milk. With the new super-absorbent nappies it's sometimes difficult to assess the urine output. Hold a fresh nappy in one hand and the used nappy in the other and compare the weights.

Q What about bottle-fed babies?

If you choose to bottle-feed, you needn't feel guilty about it; today's commercial formulas are designed to approximate the composition of breast milk, and most infants thrive and develop just as well on formula. Formula uses cow's milk or soy protein as a base but is modified to be lower in protein than cow's milk and to contain all the necessary vitamins and minerals. There is little difference between the various brands of formula, except for those prepared specifically for premature infants. Infant formulas are generally available in two forms: ready-to-use, which is the most expensive; or as a powder which is added to water. Be sure you prepare the formula exactly according to the manufacturer's instructions. Most infants take at least 150 to 180 ml per kilogram of body weight of formula each day. A baby 4 to 6 months old who gets most nutrition from formula may take a maximum of about 1200 ml per day. However, after six months of age infants start to get their daily nutrients from other foods and their intake of milk becomes much less. Infant formula should be used until six months of age and may then be transitioned onto follow-on formula, then homogenised milk as a beverage can be introduced at 12 months of age. An older baby who consumes too much milk may be missing out on other foods, which could lead to dietary imbalance and possibly iron-deficiency anaemia.

What's in that formula?

In general, formulas fall into four categories:

- cow's milk as the base
- goat's milk as the base
- soya beans as the base
- hydrolysed casein/whey formula, with the protein broken down into smaller pieces less likely to cause an allergic reaction, and does not contain lactose.

 How do I make sure my baby's bottles are sterile?

In the past most parents were careful about sterilising milk before giving it to their children, but the techniques they used may not be necessary. It is important, however, to wash your hands carefully before making up formula, and to use bottles, teats, and water that are clean and germ-free. Although many parents boil the bottles and teats, evidence suggests that fewer than 50 percent manage to prepare sterile formula. By 4 to 6 months of age, when children are putting everything in their mouths anyway, it may just be important to use clean bottles. Most parents make up one day's supply of milk and keep the bottles in the refrigerator. Most infants take formula more readily if it's warmed, although there is little evidence that they prefer it this way. Be wary of overheating formula in a microwave oven; always test the temperature before giving it to your child. Never put an infant to bed with a propped-up bottle, as the child may choke or inhale the milk; also, the constant presence of milk in the mouth encourages the growth of bacteria, producing acid and cavities.

Why are some babies put on soy-based formula?

Soy formula is not recommended for babies with a milk allergy but can be used for lactose intolerance. A *milk allergy* is a reaction to the protein in cow's milk; it may show up as a rash, coughing or wheezing, diarrhoea, or colic (see Chapter 4, 'Crying'). These symptoms should go away when the infant is taken off cow's milk. Goat's milk formula is not suitable for infants with a family history of allergy or with a cow's milk allergy, as the protein is almost identical to cow's milk.

A *lactose intolerance* is a deficiency of lactase, the enzyme that breaks down the sugar in milk (lactose). Some infants inherit a lactase deficiency; others develop it temporarily after a severe bout of gastroenteritis (intestinal flu). This may present as continued diarrhoea, or bloating, gas, and abdominal pain. These problems should disappear when the infant is taken off cow's milk products (soy does not contain lactose).

Lactose intolerance is more common in certain ethnic groups, notably those from Asia. However, it tends to be overdiagnosed; it's important to see if the symptoms actually stop completely when milk is removed from the diet, and recur when milk is reintroduced.

Note that the soy-based milks sold in many supermarkets and health food stores are not suitable for infants and should not be given in place of infant formula.

If you suspect your infant does not tolerate cow's milk based formula it is recommended that you see your doctor or an allergy specialist for advice. The Ministry of Health recommends that soy formula should only be used under the direction of a health professional for specific medical conditions.

When can I start giving my baby other foods?

Newborn infants need only breast milk or formula. On hot days, when infants lose more water by sweating – or when they are dehydrated by diarrhoea – they may take extra water between feedings. As children grow older and can indicate their thirst, they should be encouraged to drink water so they don't get into the habit of drinking too much juice or soft drink.

By 4 to 6 months of age, most infants have started infant cereals. Start with single-grain cereals with added iron, such as rice cereal. Barley, oat, or wheat can be tried later. The cereals are usually mixed with a small amount of breast milk or infant formula or water, and offered twice a day. Most parents start with a small spoonful or two, and let their infant decide how much to take. Often parents offer half the breast- or formula-feeding before the cereal, and then complete the feeding after the infant has had as much cereal as he or she wants.

Offering cereal before four months of age is neither necessary nor very successful. The natural movement of the newborn's tongue is up and forward to compress the nipple, which tends to push out solid food. It's about three or four months before infants can push food to the back of the mouth to be swallowed.

Baby teeth start to erupt around six months of age, and by that time infants are ready to eat strained or puréed foods. You can make your own with a blender or buy it in small jars. There's no need to add salt to infant foods as you might to your own.

There are few rigid rules for introducing infant foods. Cereals, fortified with iron, should probably be introduced first, but then see what your infant likes. Children have some sense of taste but appear to be less concerned about flavours than adults are. Respect your child's likes and dislikes, but encourage the sampling of many foods so he or she learns to eat a variety. Begin with bland, non-allergenic foods. Most parents start with vegetables (puréed carrots, kumara, pumpkin, marrow, potato), and later add fruits (ripe banana, apples, peaches, and pears) and meats (chicken, lamb). It's important to introduce only one new food at a time, and wait for three or four days before introducing another. That way, if your infant has an allergic reaction (a rash, diarrhoea, or vomiting), you can more easily identify the offending food.

Yellow or orange vegetables (carrots, pumpkin), which are frequently given to infants, may add a yellowish tinge to the skin, including the palms of the hands and the soles of the feet, but not to the eyes. This phenomenon is called 'carotinaemia' and is caused by the carotene in these vegetables; it has no significance and does no harm to the child.

At one year of age most children show an interest in a cup and can be weaned from the bottle. A cup, particularly one with a spout and two handles, enables the child to feed without help.

Do babies need fibre to avoid constipation?

Breast-fed infants may have infrequent stools, because breast milk is almost completely absorbed, but their stools are soft and not painful to pass; this is not constipation. On the other hand, formula-fed infants who take few solids with any fibre may be constipated, with small, pellet-like, and occasionally blood-streaked painful stools. Once children start eating more foods, make sure they get some containing fibre, including cereals.

From six months of age on, about one tooth per month erupts, until all 20 have appeared by about the age of two. During this period, when the teeth are appearing and children have more hand control, they like to put things in their mouths and chew them. You can offer soft biscuits or bread to let them feed themselves, but it's not until about one year of age that they have enough teeth to really chew. After that point they can be offered soft cooked foods that require some chewing. At this stage they want their independence; encourage them to feed themselves, no matter how messy this gets. They also develop more likes and dislikes, and some become picky eaters. There's no need to worry if your child doesn't eat at some meals; what matters is how much he or she eats over several days. This is best demonstrated by the child's ongoing weight gain.

How often should children be fed?

Most mothers who breast-feed do so whenever the child seems hungry. Most premature infants are fed every 1 to 3 hours, and full-term infants every 2 to 4 hours (six feedings a day). By the time children are sleeping through the night, they usually get five feedings a day. When solids are first introduced, they are given once or twice a day. By one year of age, most children are on three meals a day, with two or three snacks between mealtimes. Endless snacking; sugary, high-fat items; and excessive quantities of juice or soft drink should be discouraged. Children should be taught to eat when hungry and stop when satisfied.

Feeding an Older Child

In the past, doctors often gave parents strict rules about what and how much to feed their children. In most cases these rules are unnecessary; children eat according to their needs, and it's more important to offer them a balance of foods, avoiding too much added sugar, colouring, and flavour. The 1990s have seen a return to simpler, more traditional, less-processed foods. Some childhood problems, such as dental cavities from too much refined sugar or constipation from a lack of dietary fibre, may be avoided by using these more basic foods.

Some foods are dangerous because they can get stuck in the child's windpipe (trachea) or oesophagus (food passage). Raisins, grapes, and sausages are all the right size and shape to get stuck. For young children, sausages should be sliced in half or cut in small pieces. Peanuts (even crunchy peanut butter) and raw, hard, uncooked vegetables or fruit should not be offered to children under four, for the same reason.

 ### What if allergies run in the family?
If your family has a history of allergic diseases (eczema, hay fever, asthma, or food allergies), it's wise to avoid the more commonly allergenic foods. Food allergies are a greater problem for infants under one year old, since their digestive tracts allow small amounts of allergenic foods to cross the lining of the intestinal tract unchanged. If possible, breast-feed for at least a year. Delay the introduction of potentially allergenic solids such as eggs, fish, wheat and peanuts. Some children are allergic to the soy-based formulas used for children with a milk allergy; they may need hydrolysed casein/whey formula. Children under 18 months of age shouldn't be given egg-white, although they may have egg-yolk. Just because you have a particular food allergy doesn't mean your children will have the same one, so you needn't withhold the food in question; just watch closely for any indications of an allergic reaction.

 ### How can I be sure if my child has food allergies?
Many families get caught up in a pattern of avoiding all suspected foods, with the result that their children miss out on important nutrition such as calcium from milk, or iron. A child who suffers from an allergy will develop symptoms almost immediately after eating the problem food. Symptoms may be a rash, swelling of the lips, or difficulty breathing, or the diarrhoea and gas associated with cow's-milk allergy. The most common food allergies in New Zealand include milk, egg, peanuts, fish and shellfish. Skin tests may tell you what your child's *skin* reacts to, but this doesn't mean the child will react to *eating* the food. Most food allergies are diagnosed by the symptoms the child suffers after eating that food.

Introduction of weaning foods

Baby can hold head up, tongue used to move food, shows signs of chewing movements (4–6 months):

- baby rice, followed by other age-appropriate baby cereals,
- raw or cooked apple (raw apple in muslin cloth), pear, ripe banana, apricot, peaches,
- cooked and puréed potato, kūmara, pumpkin, carrot, marrow, kamokamo (marrow) and raw avocado or age appropriate commercial weaning foods.

Baby can sit, is interested in finger foods and starting to bite; some teeth are present (6–7 months):

- egg yolk,
- cooked parsnips, yams, courgettes, green beans, taro, pūhā, yams, cauliflower, broccoli, melon, nectarine, nashi pears, plums (all without skin or seeds),
- meat and chicken purées,
- toast fingers, rusks, crackers, wheat and oatmeal infant cereal – unless there is a family history of allergy,
- age-appropriate commercial weaning foods.

Baby is interested in extended range of food and varied texture – good chewing and biting (8–9 months, unless there is a strong family history of allergy, or any sign of allergy in the infant, e.g. eczema):

- fish,
- soy foods, such as tofu, tempeh, soy yoghurt; cooked silverbeet, spinach, peas and legumes, cabbage, creamed corn and raw or cooked tomatoes,
- orange, kiwifruit, pineapple, berryfruit,
- wheat e.g. bread and pasta,
- yoghurt, cottage cheese, grated cheese, ice cream,
- peanut butter (smooth).

Foods suitable from 12 months of age:

- plain pasteurised whole milk, soy milks with calcium.

If there is a strong family history of allergy, these foods should be delayed until 12 months of age:

- cheese, yoghurt, ice cream,
- fish,
- wheat cereal.

18 months to two years:

- egg white.

It is recommended that if there is a strong family history of allergy to peanuts, peanut products should not be used until after three years of age (Department of Health (UK) 1998).

Can the baby share our family's vegetarian diet?

Many children are raised on vegetarian diets, sometimes including milk (lacto-vegetarian) or eggs (ovo-vegetarian). A true 'vegan' diet, which avoids meat, milk, and eggs, can be dangerous for young children as there may be a deficiency of iron, calcium, or vitamin B_{12}. Note that a vegetarian diet shouldn't consist only of the avoidance of meat; vegetable proteins don't always have all the essential amino acids, and you may need to serve foods in specific combinations to create a complete nutritional package. Families with a long tradition of vegetarian diets, for cultural or religious reasons, know how to provide all the important dietary requirements for their children, but families just starting on a vegetarian diet are advised to talk with a dietitian about providing balanced nutrition.

 What can I do about a child who just won't eat?

Most children have good and bad days for eating. Many have favourite foods and are reluctant to eat anything else. These food preferences come and go, as long as you don't 'give in' by offering nothing but the favourites.

But a few children refuse to take any food, turning their faces away, clamping their mouths shut when food is offered, or spitting out any food you get into them. On rare occasions this is due to a physical problem, such as pain from stomach acid coming back up into the lower end of the oesophagus. More often, it's learned behaviour. Some children just don't want to eat as much as their parents would like them to, so they turn stubborn and resist whatever is offered. Children who are force-fed may find the experience painful, and refuse to co-operate. Others learn that when they refuse to eat they get more attention. The reasons for the behaviour are often complicated, but the response of the parent is generally to try to force the child to eat. *You can't force children to eat more, but you can make sure you offer foods high in energy.* There are some simple guidelines to help persuade a picky eater into having a good meal.

- Meals should be well prepared, appetising, and the kind of food the child likes, though it's not necessary to give in to every want or demand. New foods should be added gradually, in small amounts, along with food your child knows and likes. Mealtimes should be planned for times when the child is hungry. Having a child wait may disrupt his or her normal appetite.

- Offer three meals and three snacks a day, and don't offer food at other times. Nibbling or drinking between meals just spoils the appetite. Some families spend the whole day trying to get their children to eat, and then

Making mealtimes work

Nutrition and Growth

- Children don't like to sit still, but they should be encouraged to stay in a highchair or at the table. This encourages them to concentrate on eating, and prevents injuries that may happen if a child falls while eating and running.

- Watch for signs that your child is full, such as turning away from a spoon or clamping the mouth shut. Don't hover expectantly while an older child eats. Children usually eat as much as they need to keep them going, even if the amount seems small.

- Never force or bribe a child to eat; children know when they're no longer hungry. When you introduce a new food, the child may resist and turn away; rather than insisting, try again later in the meal.

- Don't use food as a reward; the impression that food equals love or approval can contribute to later eating disorders. Food also shouldn't be used as a reward for good behaviour. Good behaviour should be expected, and food, snacks, and treats should be a normal part of life.

- Offer only small amounts of food and fluids at a time. There's always more.

- Serve meals with a variety of tastes, colours, and textures, to make them more appealing. Give your child his or her own chair and place-setting, perhaps with colourful bowls and utensils.

- Remember that mood is catching. Mealtimes should be not just for eating, but for socialising with the family. Watching TV is a poor substitute for family interaction.

- Don't 'hurry along' meals. Allow young children time for play and experimentation, but stop before the mess becomes too annoying. A stress-free atmosphere promotes good lifetime food attitudes.

- Ignore food-throwing at first; it's part of normal development. Children drop things to learn the 'letting go' reflex, and how better to practise than by dumping bits of food from a highchair? Clean-up will be easier if you put newspaper or plastic sheets under the highchair. But once your child acquires the skill of letting go, don't encourage this 'game' by continually picking up dropped food. Instead, after a few throws, remove the food – the child is likely full.

- Encourage independence. Children need to practise eating, and success helps them feel good about themselves.

- Let toddlers pick food from the serving plate so they feel free to choose what and how much to eat. This helps reduce frustration during the 'no' stage. Providing limited and realistic choices encourages children to think independently. Encourage eating with a spoon so your child learns to handle utensils, but allow some finger foods to smooth the transition.

wonder why the child isn't hungry at mealtime! Snacks should be nutritious foods – fruits, vegetables, crackers and cheese or peanut butter – not biscuits, sweets or chips.

- If your child doesn't eat within a given time, such as 20 or 30 minutes, the food should be put away and nothing else offered until the next meal or snack. If your child doesn't eat what you've prepared, don't prepare something else more to his or her liking.

- Take along extra milk or a snack on your child's excursions. Find time for a healthy snack when you're out, just as you would at home.

 ## What if my child doesn't seem to be growing?

Children usually double their birthweight in the first four or five months and triple it by one year. Then their growth levels off, and many parents worry that their children don't seem to be growing to the same extent, or eating as much.

Your child's growth should be followed on a regular basis by the plunket nurse, who will measure length or height, and head circumference at each visit, comparing these with standards on a growth chart. Infants should be weighed without clothes, or nappies, on a good standardised scale. Under two years of age, length is measured lying down; after two years, standing height is measured.

The growth charts show the average weight and length/height for children at different ages, and the normal range expressed as from the third to the 97th percentile. Children usually follow the growth pattern of their parents. If the parents are tall, the child will usually be above the halfway mark (50th percentile); if the parents are short, the child's height and weight will usually be below that line. Still, whatever the family background, a child's growth should *parallel* the pattern of the growth charts.

If a child's growth is not as expected, you should discuss this with your doctor, who will want to know the height and weight of both parents and their growth patterns. Some people are small throughout childhood and go into puberty later than their peers, but then have a delayed growth spurt and reach average adult size. This very common pattern of temporary smallness can be passed on to children, and causes a lot of unnecessary worry for parents.

Your doctor will also ask about your child's health and eating, and will carry out a thorough physical exam. In most cases this will be enough to pinpoint the cause of your child's poor growth, without a lot of laboratory tests.

When children don't gain weight, it's most often because they don't eat enough good, nutritious food. The doctor may refer you to a dietitian for review of your child's eating pattern, but there's no 'magic pill' to get a child to eat. No medication has been found to stimulate children's appetite on a long-term basis. If your child doesn't eat a well-balanced diet, a supplemental vitamin may be helpful. For children who are very thin and need to gain weight, there are supplemental nutritionals available which should be given only on the advice of your doctor or dietitian.

There are also a few simple things you can do to help your child gain weight. They depend on your child's age.

- For young infants, whose diets consist primarily of milk and/or puréed foods, you can fortify the foods with supplements. This should only be done on the advice of a dietitian.

- For toddlers and older children, prepare foods that are higher in calories, and at the same time help them improve their eating behaviour.

- Fats are generally higher in calories than carbohydrates or proteins, so children who need to gain weight should be given higher-fat foods such as homogenised milk rather than two percent or skim, butter or margarine, cheese, cream, and peanut butter. Butter, margarine, salad oils and dressings, yoghurt, sour cream, or cheese sauces can be added to other foods. But sweets such as confectionary, cakes, and biscuits may satisfy children sooner than more nutritious complex-carbohydrate food such as bread, pastas, potatoes, rice, or other cereals, so that in the end they eat *less*.

- Try making sandwiches with two slices of meat plus cheese; adding small pieces of cooked meat, poultry, or tofu to macaroni, omelettes, quiches, soups, or salads; spreading peanut butter on sandwiches, muffins, crackers, or pancakes; and serving nuts or seeds as snacks or added to ice cream or yoghurt. (Nuts should not be given to children under four as they may be accidentally inhaled into the lungs.)

Overweight Children

Infants and toddlers have different body proportions than adults, with larger trunks and shorter legs. They may thus appear to be fat or 'chubby' when they are normal, healthy children. However, some children do gain too much weight for their age and height. There is good evidence that obesity tends to run in families, both because of genetic factors and because children learn patterns of overeating and underexercising from their families.

Obesity is seen most commonly in one-year-olds, preschoolers, and young adolescents. It's usually the result of two factors: the children eat more than necessary, and are less active and don't burn off the energy they take in. If a child has a tendency to obesity, it's easier to deal with it early, before the child is grossly overweight. Weight-loss programmes for children have generally been unsuccessful unless the *child* is highly motivated to lose weight.

If you feel your infant or toddler is overweight, talk to your doctor before making major changes in the child's diet, to be certain the child is truly over-weight according to the growth chart; he or she may not be overweight at all. You have more control over what your child eats at this age, so you can help your child develop a diet that doesn't include high-energy foods. (Initially this may be more useful than trying to control the *amount* the child eats.) After one year of age, overweight children should be given reduced fat milk rather than homogenised milk, smaller amounts of food, and foods with lower fat content.

There is little evidence that obesity in young children predisposes them to obesity in adulthood. There is also little evidence that early obesity predisposes children to weight-related diseases such as atherosclerosis (hardening of the arteries), heart disease, or diabetes in adulthood. On the other hand, we know that these diseases also tend to run in families. If your family has a history of obesity and these related conditions, it's prudent to try to manage your child's weight problem as early as possible.

 What about an older overweight child?

Avoid offering more food than the child wants, and don't offer food outside of regular meal and snack times. Snacks should be nutritious vegetables, fruits, crackers or breads. Juice, soft drink, and milk can provide a lot of energy; offer them in moderation. A child who is just thirsty should be given water.

Discourage your child from eating too much just before bedtime, which can set up bad habits. If physical activity and exercise are a normal pattern for your family, your child will readily copy your example.

If an older child is concerned about actual overweight, it may be best for the child to set the goal of maintaining present weight. As the child grows taller, the weight will be more appropriately distributed, with less fat. If the child wants to maintain weight, or even lose weight, it's probably best to encourage smaller amounts of low-fat foods rather than follow a specific weight-loss diet designed for adults. Children should avoid overeating, second helpings, eating when they're bored rather than hungry, and eating after dinner. They should drink reduced fat milk, and avoid excessive amounts of high energy foods, e.g. peanut butter, potato chips, french fries and fatty foods. Snacks should be nutritious or lower in energy: fruits and vegetables, crackers, popcorn without butter or margarine. Biscuits and chips should be avoided.

A child who wants to lose weight can benefit from regular exercise such as walking or cycling. Twenty to 30 minutes of exercise a day will burn up more energy than reading, watching television or computer activities.

 ### What about an overweight teenager?

As children get into their teens, their behaviour – including eating – is often influenced more by their peers and by advertising than by their parents. They want to 'follow the crowd' and do what their friends do. For girls who are self-conscious about their weight, this may mean skipping meals, avoiding certain foods, or experimenting with diets. For boys who are concerned about their athletic ability, this may mean taking food, protein, or vitamin and mineral supplements. Some teens, especially those who are concerned about their weight or have a busy schedule, start to skip meals, particularly breakfast. Children need food energy for the day's activities. Breakfast is probably the most important meal, and should not be skipped.

Some teenagers stop drinking milk, or stop eating meat. Milk is a major source of calcium required for bone growth, and is very important during puberty. Meat provides a valuable source of protein, vitamins, and iron. Inadequate intakes of calcium and iron are not uncommon in young people today. If your teenager wants to avoid certain foods, he or she should seek advice from a dietitian or your doctor.

Teenagers also spend a lot of time watching television and eating snacks. Again, it's not easy to tell them how to behave, but even teens tend to follow their parents' example.

As a parent, you need to be aware of what your child is or is not eating. It's pointless to force or nag or tell teens what to do, but you can help them seek good nutritional advice from your doctor, from magazines and books, or from nutritional counsellors. Remember, bad eating habits are easier to prevent than to correct. You can help your children get off to a good start by showing them moderate, balanced eating habits, and a healthy lifestyle with regular exercise.

CHAPTER 13

Safety at Home and Away

njuries are the leading health problem of children in New Zealand, resulting in approximately 130 deaths and 10,500 hospital admissions per year among children younger than 15 years of age. More than half of all childhood deaths result from injuries, exceeding deaths due to cancer; congenital anomalies (problems present at birth); and diseases of the nervous system, heart, and respiratory system. Deaths are only the tip of the iceberg. It is estimated that for every injury death, about 80 people are admitted to hospital and several hundred are treated at emergency departments.

Motor vehicle traffic crashes are the leading causes of injury death among pre-schoolers (less than five years) in New Zealand, followed by suffocation/choking and drowning. The leading cause of injury hospitalisation in the under-five age group is falls, followed by (accidental) poisoning and burns or scalds.

Motor vehicle collisions are the leading cause of injury death for children aged 5 to 14. Almost 65 percent of these are passengers in motor vehicles and 34 percent are pedestrian deaths. One in 10 school-age children who die in collisions are bicyclists. The leading cause of injury hospitalisation for this age group is falls, followed by cycling injuries. After one year of age, boys suffer more of almost every kind of injury than girls.

Often these injuries are described as 'accidents', which suggests that the harm could not have been expected, and therefore could not have been prevented. The more we understand about how injuries happen, the more we recognise that there are recurring patterns that can be anticipated, and changed. We should therefore abandon the word 'accident' and begin to consider most injuries preventable.

Why might my child be at risk of injuries?

There are many factors that make a child vulnerable to one kind of injury or another. One is the child's development and temperament: children are curious, spontaneous and exploratory by nature and like to imitate behaviours they observe in others around them, whether this be brothers and sisters, friends, or adults. Some behaviours or situations are likely to pose particular threats to the safety of young children more than older individuals. Crossing a busy traffic-congested street would be one example. Given normal patterns of development, children are sometimes not fully capable of perceiving, understanding and responding safely to this potentially hazardous and complex situation. Yet another factor that places a child at risk is his/her environment, both physical and social. By and large, children live in an adult world. Many private and public places do not account for the needs and capabilities of young people. These situations can therefore be particular hazards for unsupervised children. The need to supervise and monitor children constantly, in turn, places considerable strain on busy families living in poorly resourced and unsafe environments.

What should I be doing about these risks?

There are many steps parents can take on their own. While supervising children is important, it is particularly important to take what steps possible to make the environment children grow up in as safe as possible. 'Child-proofing' homes, staying aware of the latest safety developments, and generally thinking ahead to the risks their children may encounter are some key steps.

There are also steps that require the involvement of others. There are many things that government and local body authorities can do to promote the safety of all citizens. In general, a community that is safe for its children is safe for individuals of all ages. This requires political will, commitment and resources.

A role that parent groups can be very effective in is advocating for proven safety standards, and encouraging the enforcement of mandatory standards, e.g., for nursery furniture and playground equipment. Another area that can make a difference is responding to community concerns. Are there dangerous sites in your neighbourhood that attract children? Should there be traffic lights or a pedestrian crossing at a certain intersection, or more spot-checks for drinking drivers? Consider what happens after an injury occurs. Are your fire and ambulance services well equipped? Could volunteers be trained for community emergencies? Does your local hospital need better facilities? You may want to get involved in a parents' coalition, community injury prevention programme, school-based forum and/or KidSafe Week coalition to tackle questions like these. You could also contact the local city council, public health office or health service provider to find out more about programmes in your area.

This chapter provides advice on some steps you can take to reduce the likelihood of injury for your child/children. While this may seem a tedious list of dos and don'ts and it does not guarantee your child grows up injury-free, his/her likelihood of experiencing a serious injury should be considerably reduced. With increasing knowledge and information on more effective ways to prevent injury, guidelines and laws promoting child safety in New Zealand are also likely to change. It is therefore important to be aware of these and put into practice recommendations that may apply to your family's needs. Lastly, it is likely that financial assistance may be available for some potentially expensive products and home modifications. Where relevant, discuss these with your health provider, Plunket nurse, Housing New Zealand or Work and Income New Zealand.

Motor Vehicle Crashes

How can I protect my child in a car crash?

Motor-vehicle occupant injuries are the leading cause of death for older children and adolescents, and a common cause of death for children at younger ages. Fatal or serious non-fatal injuries usually result when a child with no seatbelt or car safety seat is thrown against the interior of the car, such as the windscreen, dashboard, or front seat. Infants held in arms are as likely to be seriously injured or killed as unrestrained children. In a crash, it is physically impossible for an adult to hold onto an infant.

It is strongly recommended that children always travel in the back seat. This is particularly the case for young infants in rear facing infant car seats, children travelling in cars fitted with air bags, and those travelling in cars which don't have a car seat or seatbelt for children to wear.

The best way to protect your child in a car crash is to obey the law and 'buckle them in'. New Zealand law requires that children under five years of age always be in approved child restraints (car seats) when they travel in a motor vehicle. Children 5 to 7 years old must use a child restraint or seatbelt if there is one available. Children aged 8 to 14 years must use a seatbelt if available. It is the driver's responsibility to make sure children are buckled into appropriate restraints.

Car restraints do more than secure children in the car to make it less likely they hit the inside of the vehicle. They help spread the forces of the crash over the strongest parts of the child's body. But restraints must be installed following the manufacturer's guidelines. Incorrect installation is a very common problem and decreases the child's protection.

The right type of car restraint for your child will change as the child grows. The following is a guide that will help you choose and install the most appropriate car restraint for your child/children.

Choosing a car restraint suitable for your child

When selecting a child car seat make sure that you get one that:

- suits your child's size and weight (see guide below),

- can be correctly fitted in your car. Because of the different shapes of vehicle seats, some car seats may fit better than others. Take the car seat out to your car and try it,

- is approved by the Standards Association of New Zealand. Look for the 'S' mark when buying a seat.

Choosing a car restraint suitable for your child

Age	Type
Under six months (less than 9 kg)	Rear facing infant seat
Birth to four years (up to 18kg)	Birth to four years seat
Six months to four years (9kg to 18kg)	Child seat
Two years to eight years (14kg to 32kg)	Booster Seat
Two years to eight years	Child Harness
Over eight years	Adult seat belt

Second-hand car restraints

Many second-hand car seats sold through local advertising have been found to be unsafe. It is recommended that if you are buying a second-hand car seat or going to use one passed on by family or friends, you check it carefully for the following:

- are you sure the seat has not been involved in a crash or been otherwise damaged?

- does it have a label stating it meets a standard accepted for sale in New Zealand?

- is there an instruction book with the seat?

- does the seat have all its parts, no fraying on the harness and does the buckle work well?

If in doubt about the safety of a second-hand seat, don't buy it. Don't sell a car seat you know is not safe for use.

Further information on car restraints

There are several sources of information to assist you when buying or renting a child car seat. The Plunket Society co-ordinates a national scheme which offers advice and a rental scheme. Many regions also have schemes co-ordinated by Maori and Pacific health providers. Information and advice can also be obtained from the SafeKids Information Centre (see contact information at the end of this book). In some cases, Work and Income New Zealand (WINZ) may be able to provide financial assistance for families wishing to buy car seats.

How can I protect my child as a pedestrian?

Pedestrian injuries are the leading cause of death in children 5 to 9 years of age. Because the force of the impact is so great, severe multiple injuries are common, including head injuries. Older children are more at risk on public roads, typically while enroute to a particular destination, such as school or the local dairy. Younger children, especially toddlers, are at risk of being run over in their driveways, particularly where the driveway is shared. Preventing pedestrian injury requires separating children from cars, slowing traffic in areas where children tend to cross the street, providing adult supervision for children unable to make safe decisions about street crossing, and training older children in street-crossing strategies. As a general rule, children under eight years should cross streets only with adult supervision, and those aged under 10 years, should not cross major streets without adult supervision.

Both here and overseas there is a trend for more children to be picked up and dropped off at school. This frequently creates an unsafe situation for our children. There are some common sense rules parents can follow to help in this situation:

- always set a good example to your children when crossing the road – this will help ensure their safety when you aren't there,

- walk to the school gate to drop off or collect your child – always hold on to little hands,

- never call out from across the road – excited children forget to look for traffic,

- take extreme care when pulling into driveways close to the school – child pedestrians can be unpredictable and unaware of your presence.

What about bicycle safety?

Bicycling is very popular among school-age children. It is estimated that around 87 percent of children aged 8 to 14 years in New Zealand own a bicycle and that three quarters are riding at least once a week. Bicycle injuries usually occur when children either fall off their bikes or collide with fixed objects (e.g., curb or a tree) or motor vehicles. About 15 percent of bike injuries are serious resulting in death or longer-term disability; these are mostly due to head injury. A range of strategies can help protect children from serious bicycle injuries:

- all bicyclists must wear helmets (see following section);

- the New Zealand Police, the Land Transport Safety Authority and Safekids advise that children should not ride on the road under 10 years of age unless they are accompanied by an adult. Ideally, children under 10 should ride only with adult supervision, and off the street;

- skills training: this is important in all contexts but particular skills children riding in traffic need include: riding single-file in a straight line, without swerving or moving between parked cars; stopping at all inter-sections; using hand signals when stopping and turning; checking over the shoulder when turning. Remember that your child is unlikely to obey safety rules if you yourself disregard them;

- children, in general, should be discouraged from riding cycles after dark; older children riding with their parents must have front and rear lights and reflective clothing when riding after dark, as should their parents;

- make sure you and your child know basic bike maintenance and the importance of keeping the bike cleaned, oiled and checked regularly, with particular attention to the brakes;

- parents should be aware of where children ride bikes and check that the location is safe given the child's age and development.

Bike helmets provide protection

Studies suggest that a bicycle helmet may reduce the risk of head injury by 85 percent. In New Zealand all cyclists are required by law to wear an approved safety helmet when cycling. An 'approved' helmet is one that bears an approved to New Zealand Standards ('S') mark.

Bike helmets are specially designed to withstand high-impact collisions. Helmets should cover the top of the forehead, sitting not too far forward or too far backward. The straps should be snug without pinching and should be easy to do up. Take care not to buy a helmet that is too small or too large. While padding is available to insert in bike helmets, excessive padding to make a helmet fit firmly may affect its performance. It is important that a bike helmet is fitted by a person who knows how. Helmet retailers and cycle shops usually have staff who can do this for you. A helmet should not be used if it has been mistreated, dropped or involved in a crash. Even if it looks undamaged, it may have lost much of its strength. Helmets should be replaced every three years.

At what age should I buy my child a bicycle?

Consider allowing your child to ride a two-wheeled bike at about five or six years of age. When buying a bike, go with your child to an approved dealer and match the child to the bike. In particular, look for a safety standard label on the bike and check that the bike is the right size, using the following guidelines:

- sitting on the seat with both hands on the handlebars, your child must be able to place the balls of both feet on the round;

- straddling the centre bar, your child should be able to keep both feet flat on the ground with about 2.5 cm (an inch) clearance between crotch and bar; and

- the child should be able to grasp the hand brakes and apply enough pressure to stop the bike.

All of the recommendations above are just as important if you are getting a second-hand bike or your child acquires one passed on from another child (e.g., older brother or sister).

Preventing the tragedy of fire: install and maintain smoke alarms

How often have you heard about children dying in a house fire because there was no smoke alarm, or because the alarm's battery had been removed or had gone dead? Many people mean to install alarms but 'don't get around to it'. If you don't already have enough alarms, it should be high on your list of priorities for injury prevention. Housing New Zealand has also made a commitment to installing smoke alarms in rental properties managed by them.

If you're not sure how many alarms you need, check the alarm instructions, or consult your fire department. Alarms should be checked once a month, and it's wise to change the batteries once a year – pick a day and make it a ritual (let older children help, to reinforce their awareness of fire safety).

Install a fire extinguisher in the kitchen, and in any other area where fire is particularly likely (such as the garage or workshop). Check it regularly to be sure it's still charged. Everyone old enough to handle the extinguishers should know how to remove them from their mountings and use them.

Get pamphlets on fire safety from your local fire department and teach your children what to do in a fire. Practise fire drill as a game. If any parts of your home have limited access (such as upper bedrooms with a single staircase), consult your fire department about emergency escape equipment.

Even if you never have a fire, the safety you practise at home will set a valuable example for your children.

Injuries at Home

While injuries in and around home are significant for children of all ages, they are especially common for those under five years. The most common forms of home injury deaths are suffocation, fires and burns, and drowning. Falls are the leading cause of non-fatal home injuries. Keeping children safe at home involves two key strategies: developing safer family practices and creating a safer home environment.

How can I prevent injuries in the kitchen?

Whenever possible, keep toddlers out of the kitchen – especially during meal preparation, when hazards are greater and you may be too preoccupied to supervise closely. If necessary, provide a safe zone, for example a playpen. In addition:

- avoid small refrigerator magnets, which can be a choking hazard;

- don't place an infant or older child on the kitchen bench or counter top;

- don't place an infant in an infant seat or 'bouncinet' on a bench or other elevated area;

- keep rubbish secured behind a latched door;

- rearrange storage areas so that dangerous equipment, cleaning compounds, and foods are kept in upper shelves, cabinets and drawers, and safe items in lower shelves, cabinets and drawers;

- if dangerous items must be contained in cabinets and drawers the child can reach, install child-guard latches for these areas;

- set aside one cabinet or kitchen cupboard for safe items that the child can explore;

- keep knives and other sharp objects away from counter edges, and when not in use store where children cannot reach them;

- clean up spills immediately to avoid slipping.

 How can I prevent scalds and burns?

- If a playpen is located in the kitchen, keep it well away from the stove;

- don't carry hot liquid when you're carrying a child;

- don't place hot items at the edge of the counter or table;

- use the back burners on the stove when possible;

- turn pot handles inward on the stove;

- keep your child away from ovens or other appliances that may be hot on the outside;

- never leave an appliance cord plugged into an outlet when the cord is disconnected from the appliance;

- keep appliances and electrical cords (e.g., of kettle, toaster, iron) out of reach and away from the edges of counters;

- avoid heating formula or food in a microwave, as it may heat unevenly and scald a child's mouth;

- if you must use a microwave, mix the food thoroughly after heating, allow to stand for five or more minutes and test the food or drink before serving;

- use fireguards with all fires and heaters making sure fingers can't be burned through bars;

- keep ashtrays, cigarettes, matches and lighters out of sight and reach;

- reduce the hot water temperature (see section on safety in bathtubs);

- dress children in clothing that is loose fitting. Be aware that cotton material burns very easily. Check nightwear for low fire-risk labels.

 Do I have to do anything in the living room or family room?
Although these rooms may look safe, when children are being playful or exploring they can easily hurt themselves. Therefore:

- make sure all furniture is stable;

- check that handles and knobs are secure, and large enough that they don't present a choking hazard;

- cover sharp edges of furniture, for example, coffee tables, with corner guards;

- avoid glass-topped tables;

- keep window-blind and curtain cords out of reach so children can't strangle themselves;

- avoid falls from windows by installing window guards or locking devices that won't allow a window to open more than 10 cm (four inches);

- make sure children don't run near glass doors and windows. Put bright stickers or strips on all large areas of glass;

- store all alcohol in a child resistant cupboard.

 What should I do about electrical cords and appliances?

- Use as few electrical cords as possible, and move them behind furniture so they can't be chewed or tugged. Avoid using extension cords.

- Install safety switches.

 138

- Cover electrical outlets with shields, and place heavy furniture in front of them.

- Don't leave a lamp without a bulb.

- Keep hot light bulbs out of your child's reach.

- Install protective barriers on fireplaces, heaters, stoves, and radiators.

- If at all possible, avoid using space heaters. If this cannot be avoided, make sure the heater turns off automatically if toppled, and turn it off when adults are out of the room or asleep. Keep all heaters out of reach of children.

 Are playpens and baby walkers safe?

A playpen may be used as a safe area, but check that it has fine mesh sides with openings less than half a centimetre, or vertical bars or slats with gaps that are 50 mm to 85 mm wide. The playpen should always be fully open so that it can't collapse and so that there are no spaces between the mattress and the sides. It is important to ensure that all slats are vertical to prevent a child from climbing out.

Baby walkers should be avoided. The use of baby walkers can slow child development, and most importantly, are associated with an unacceptably high risk of injury. Injuries are particularly likely when baby-walkers are used close to open doorways, stairs, on uneven floors or floors with rugs or unsecured carpets. Children in baby-walkers, particularly if unattended, could get close to and be hurt by objects on tables, hot liquids, ovens, space heaters and fireplaces.

 What about the dining room?

Follow the same precautions as in the living room. In addition:

- keep heavy or fragile objects out of reach;

- don't use long tablecloths that overhang the table;

- be sure the highchair has a wide base so it won't easily topple over;

- keep the child strapped in when he or she is in the highchair, and ensure the straps are working properly;

- never leave the child unattended in the highchair.

139

And the bedroom?

Take the same measures as in the living room. Also:

- do not place cushions or pillows in the cot or wherever infants sleep;

- never let infants sleep on an adult bed, because they can become trapped between the bed and wall and suffocate;

- don't leave an infant unattended on a changing table;

- use covered waste-baskets, or don't place hazardous items in an open waste-basket (for example, plastic bags, small or sharp items including buttons, rubber bands and balloons);

- use open bins, baskets and shelves for toy storage; avoid toy chests, particularly those with heavy lids that can snap shut on young hands. Drill holes in the body of toy boxes that are closed;

- keep window-blind or curtain cords out of reach; don't place a crib, bassinet, playpen, chair or bed within reach of a window-blind or curtain cord;

- avoid falls from windows by installing window guards or locking devices that won't allow a window to open more than 10 cm (four inches);

- do not keep childrens' medications by their bedside table;

- make sure the paint and fillings of the toys aren't toxic. Infants and young children often lick or bite toys and it is important to ensure they won't be poisoned or hurt by this;

- check that soft toys are fire resistant and that the fillings can't come out easily because the child could choke on it;

- it is not safe for young children (especially those under three years of age) to have toys with detachable parts. Children can swallow these parts and choke.

 How can I be sure my child's bed is safe?

Your baby or small child may spend a lot of time in their cot and it is therefore important to make sure this is a safe space. When buying a cot make sure it meets the standards recommended by the Ministry of Consumer Affairs in New Zealand (AS/NZS2172). Always read the manufacturer's instructions, and follow them when assembling and using the cot. The Ministry of Consumer Affairs has published checklists to help families when choosing and using cots (see appendix) and has introduced a mandatory standard for new and second hand cots.

Apart from the structure of the cot, there are some other important issues to consider in using a cot.

- Never leave the rails down when the baby is in the cot.

- Don't hang any cot toys within reach and remove toys strung across the crib when the child is beginning to push up on hands and knees, or is five months of age.

- Don't leave large toys or other objects in the cot – small children may pile these up to climb out; likewise, do not place the cot close to other furniture which could provide a foothold to allow a child to climb out.

- Place a rug or carpet under the cot.

- Make sure the cot is not close to a window with curtains or blind cords, and that there are no toys or cot bumper pads tied with long strings or ribbons; these can strangle a small child.

- Keep the cot well away from power points and do not use electric blankets in the cot.

- Do not leave plastic wrapping, bags or sheets on the mattress as these can suffocate a baby. Always remove the manufacturer's plastic bag from the cot mattress before use.

- Don't put a pillow in the cot because this can suffocate your baby.

Second-hand cots may have been painted with lead-base paint. If your baby chews on lead-base paint, they can get sick very quickly. Ask your plunket nurse or local plunket clinic for details on how to check if the paint is lead-based – this is a free service.

Toddler beds should ideally have guard (safety) rails and should be placed at least half a metre (two feet) from windows, heating vents, radiators, wall lamps, curtains and window-blind cords.

The use of bunk beds, while popular, are discouraged by many health professionals because of the risk young children have of falling out of them. Children under six should not sleep in the top bunk, and vigorous or rough play should not be allowed on either bunk. If bunk beds are unavoidable, they should have guard (safety) rails next to the wall and at both ends on the upper and lower bunks, and on the outer side on the upper bunk. The guard-rails should extend at least 13 cm (five inches) above the mattress, and the mattress should sit on cross supports of wood slats, metal straps, or sturdy wires. To prevent the risk of a child getting trapped, attach additional boards to the bunk bed to close up any space more than 9 cm (three inches) wide between the lower edge of the guard rails and the upper edge of the bed frame.

 What about safety in the bathroom?

It is important to keep children out of the bathroom when they're not using it by keeping the door securely closed. Don't have any inside locks that you can't open from the outside. In addition:

- keep the toilet lid closed;

- make sure nappy buckets and any other liquid containers are closed or covered;

- use non-slip bathmats;

- use a covered wastebasket;

- store electricals (i.e., hairdryers, electrical shavers, etc.) safely and away from water when not in use;

- keep medications, cleaning and toilet products and other harmful items out of sight and out of reach; wherever possible use a locked cabinet;

- wherever possible, get medications in child-resistant containers;

- keep the phone number of the National Poisons Information Centre handy.

 Are there special precautions for the bathtub?

Never leave an infant or child unattended in the water. Children can drown in as little as 4 cm of water and must be supervised at all times. If you're bathing an infant or child, ignore all other interruptions; don't leave 'for a moment' to answer the door or telephone. Never leave water in the tub when it's not in use. Also:

- be sure the bath bottom is slip-proof;

- keep electrical appliances away from water, don't leave them plugged in;

- don't leave soap and shampoo on the edge of the bath.

The best way to protect your child from hot water scalds is to make sure the household water comes out of the tap at no higher than 50° C (120° F). Contact with hot water at a temperature of 50–55° C usually allows one minute before causing a serious burn to a child. There are three options to achieve 'safe' hot water:

- install a tempering valve;

- turn down your hot water cylinder;

- install temperature-limiting taps and shower mixers.

   A few other things that assist are:

- turning on the cold tap before the hot one, and turning off the hot tap before the cold one;

- where possible, using a single tap rather than separate hot and cold ones;

- always testing the water temperature before placing the child in the bath.

Hot water safety is a complex issue. For further information, please contact the Safekids Information Centre (see resources list).

Do I need to do anything in hallways and on stairs?

Children are frequently injured by a fall down stairs. It is recommended that gates or stair guards should be put in at the top and bottom of the stairs when your infant begins to crawl. When buying a safety barrier to block access to stairs, make sure it meets New Zealand standards (see specifications at the end of this chapter). Keep stairs and hallways clear of objects and check that both stairs and hallways are well lit at night. Clean up spills immediately to avoid slipping.

What about other parts of the house?

There are many substances that are toxic to children kept in sheds, garages and other outside areas. Wherever they are kept, ensure all substances such as cleaners, fertilisers, pesticides, car polishes, petrol and oil are kept out of the reach of children in a locked cabinet or a child resistant container. In the laundry keep detergents, bleach, and other products in a cabinet out of reach. Keep children away from standing water in buckets, nappy pails, and other containers. In addition:

- keep all doors and screens secured and mark all glass doors with tape or pictures to avoid children walking into them;

- do not keep guns in your home. If you must keep one, have it locked up, inaccessible, and unloaded, and store the bullets in a separate location.

Water Safety

Drowning is a major cause of death in children. About half of all drownings occur in lakes, ponds, rivers, and oceans, and half in residential swimming pools. Drowning rates are highest for children under five. Young children don't understand the dangers of falling into water, and may not be able to call for help. Most young victims drown during short periods of time (often less than five minutes) when no adult is supervising. While precautions can help make children safe around water nothing can replace adult supervision at all times. In case something does happen, you and anyone else who cares for your child should learn basic water-rescue techniques and cardiopulmonary resuscitation (CPR). Any child who may have inhaled water should have immediate medical attention; even if the child seems fine, the water may have caused lung damage.

 How can I make swimming and swimming pools safer for my child?

It is estimated that effective barriers around swimming pools would prevent up to 70 percent of pool drownings. The Swimming Pool Act 1987 was designed to protect young children from drowning in unfenced swimming pools. It requires all privately owned swimming pools and spa pools to be fenced. The fence must surround the pool and the area directly around it. The standard of fencing required is set out in the Building Code. For more detailed information contact your local council and Water Safe New Zealand.

Swimming lessons may provide a false sense of security for both parent and child. The emphasis on teaching children needs to be on developing safe attitudes and practices around water.

Boating injuries are more common among young adults and adults than

---

Plan for the best, prepare for the worst

no matter what precautions you take, you should still be prepared to deal with injuries.

- Keep emergency numbers (e.g. ambulance / fire service, emergency health provider) within handy reach of the telephone.

- Keep a first-aid kit at home, in your car, and anywhere else you're likely to need one and know the indications for its use.

- Take a first-aid course that includes CPR, and encourage babysitters and others who care for your child to do the same. For more information on first-aid courses, and specific advice for life-threatening emergencies, see Chapter 18, 'Emergency First Aid'. You could also contact your local 'Citizens Advice Bureau', public library or local chapter of the Order of St John for information regarding courses.

- In the event of an injury, contact your health provider or if necessary, the after-hours or emergency health service.

---

children. The two most effective precautions are using personal flotation devices (or safety jackets) of the right type and size for age of child, and not operating a boat under the influence of alcohol.

Playground Injuries

Most playground injuries are minor, but up to one-quarter may require a hospital assessment and usually involve head injuries and broken bones. Most playground injuries are caused by falls from playground equipment (especially climbing equipment) to the surface. Concrete and asphalt surfaces are more dangerous than sand and similar artificial surfaces. Equipment should be inspected for projecting bolts and sharp edges, as well as overall maintenance. Equipment should be placed so that collisions are unlikely. While there are playground standards operating in New Zealand which aim to promote the safety of children using these facilities, you may wish to evaluate the safety of your local public and school playgrounds for yourself.

How dangerous is roller-blading (or in-line skating)?

Most childhood roller-blading (or in-line skating) injuries occur in children 10 to 14 years of age, on roads and sidewalks. Almost half of these result in broken bones or dislocations, while the remainder consist of lesser injuries such as sprains, cuts, bruises, and scrapes. The child's hand or arm is most often injured. Children should wear a helmet, kneepads, elbow pads, and wrist pads. They should only skate in traffic-free areas such as rinks, parks and playgrounds.

Key contacts and resources for child safety are listed in the 'Where to find support and information' chapter at the back of this book.

Appendix

Safety recommendations and checklists for selected products in New Zealand (as of June 2000)

As standards, legislation and safety recommendations are updated on the basis of new information, readers are advised to contact Safekids or other listed resources for up-to-date information.

Cots

- All edges smooth and rounded.

- The cot is more than half a metre deep – measure from the top of the mattress to the top of the cot side.

- The gaps between the bars in the cot sides and ends are 50–85 mm wide.

- The space between the mattress and the cot sides or ends is less than 25 mm.

- The drop side can be securely locked.

- Nothing sticks into or out of the cot – i.e., no screws, nails or other parts of the cot.

- The cot will not collapse when it is being used or moved.

- The base of the cot does not sag or collapse when pushed down.

- There are no gaps that could trap a baby's head or arms:
  - gaps 30–50 mm wide can trap legs or arms;
  - gaps bigger than 85 mm wide can trap a baby's head;
  - a baby can fall through gaps wider than 95 mm.

- The dropside can't be opened by a child.

- The corner posts don't stick up over the cot end more than 8 mm.

- There are no bars, ledges or other footholds that a child can use to climb out of the cot.

- There are no transfers, counting beads or name tiles on the cot.

Portable Cots and Play-yards

- Ask the shop assistant to show you how to fold and put it up.

- Make sure the catches lock firmly.

- Check that the mattress fits snugly.

- Does it have a removable base? If so, check that the base can be firmly secured.

- Does it have bars? If so, check that spaces between bars are between 50 mm and 85 mm.

- Ask the shop assistant if the

product complies with a safety standard. The cot or play-yard should meet the standards AS/NZS2172 (for wooden cots) and AS/NZS2195 (for folding cots).

Playpens

- Height: the top edge of the play-pen floor is 600 mm or more from the floor.

- Gaps between the bars or slats are between 50–85 mm wide.

- Bars or slats are vertical to prevent a child from climbing out.

Safety Barriers

- Safety barriers should meet the standards AS1879 or NZS5843.

- Height of the barrier is at least 750 mm from the floor.

- Bars or slats are vertical to prevent child from climbing out.

- Gaps between the bars or slats are between 50–85 mm wide.

Child Restraints

- Standards Association of New Zealand. Look for the 'S' mark when buying a seat. See the information in this chapter for further details.

- Safe restraints will have passed one of the following standards:

- New Zealand Standard 5411 (Displays an 'S' mark);
- Australian Standard 1754 (Displays a tick);
- Australian & New Zealand Standard AS/NZS1754;
- United States Standard FMVSS213;
- European Standard ECE44 (Displays an 'e').

Swimming Pool Fencing

Relevant legislation:

- Swimming Pool Act 1987.

- Building Act 1991.

Requirements:

- gap between ground and fence/gates is not more than 100 mm;

- gaps in fencing cladding not more than 100 mm;

- rail spacing to be 900 mm;

- mesh/net openings:
  - 1.2 m fence – not more than 10 mm,
  - 1.8 m fence – not more than 50 mm;

- gate must open outwards;

- gates automatically shut with latches;

- gate latch must be self-locking;

- ranch sliders must have top bolts;

- steps to be removable to Para-type pools (if applicable);

- if pools are 1.2 m above ground, the sides should be smooth and vertical e.g., Para-type pools.

Fire Safety: Smoke Alarms

- Fire Service recommends only smoke alarms which have certification under the following manufacturing specifications:
  – ANSI/UL217;
  – BS 5446;
  – ULC S531.
  – Buy smoke alarms that are labelled as complying with US, Canadian, British or Australian Standards.
  – When mounting smoke alarms, refer to manufacturer's instructions or NZ 4514: 1989 The Installation of Smoke Alarms.
  – Install in centre of ceiling. If not possible, then install at least 300 mm from any corner or wall. If they are on a wall, put them 300 mm from the ceiling.

Standards

For more information on safety standards, please contact:

Standards Association of New Zealand
115 The Terrace
Private Bag 2439, Wellington
Ph: 04 498 5990; Fax 04 498 5994
E-mail: snz@standards.co.nz

Ministry of Consumer Affairs
PO Box 11473, Wellington
Ph: 04 474 2750; Fax 04 473 9400
E-mail: mcainfo@mca.govt.nz
Website: www.consumer-ministry.govt.nz

In addition to the above, you could contact your local Public Health Office or City Council to get information and contact details for:

- local iwi providers supporting safe community and health programmes;

- Pacific and other migrant resource groups;

- local community injury prevention programmes operating in your area.

CHAPTER 14

Diseases and Medical Conditions

• •

A full listing of the diseases and conditions that may affect children is beyond the scope of this book, but the following are problems frequently encountered, or of particular concern. They are presented alphabetically for ease of reference. Topics covered are:

- asthma;
- bronchiolitis;
- chickenpox (varicella);
- colds (viral upper-respiratory infections);
- croup;
- diphtheria;
- fifth disease (erythema infectiosum);
- haemophilus influenzae B (epiglottitis);

- hepatitis;
- measles;
- mumps;
- pertussis (whooping cough);
- pneumonia;
- roseola;
- rubella (German measles);
- scarlet fever and strep throat;
- tetanus.

Asthma
• • • • • • • • • • • •

Approximately 5 to 10 percent of children have at least mild asthma at some period in their lives. It's a leading cause of chronic illness in childhood, one of the most common reasons for admission to a children's hospital, and a major cause of school absenteeism. Fortunately, many children outgrow it.

Asthma is characterised by recurrent bouts of wheezing, coughing, and shortness of breath. The airways are 'hyperactive' – they react more than normal to various stimuli, and respond with narrowing and inflammation. The stimuli include such things as smoke, dust and paint, exercise, colds, and even cold air. The most common offending agent in young children is a cold. Second-hand smoke is another common trigger, especially in infants. One of the greatest causes of asthma in New Zealand is allergy to house dust mites. Older children are more likely to be allergic, reacting to pets, pollens, and moulds; humidifiers are a source of moulds and must be cleaned regularly. The season of the year is significant: asthma which occurs in early spring suggests tree allergies as a trigger, late spring and summer suggests grasses, and mid-February to the first frost may suggest ragweed. Emotional factors are rarely important in causing childhood asthma.

 ### When and how does asthma first appear?

The vast majority of asthmatic children develop symptoms by age five. The typical case is a young child who develops a cold, and several days later begins to cough, wheeze, and breathe quickly. You may hear a wheeze when the child breathes out. The child may be short of breath, with the lower ribs sucking in on each breath. Another common example is the child who wheezes and coughs with exercise, especially in a cold environment. Some children never wheeze but develop a cough, usually dry and non-productive, when exposed to triggers. These are the children who have a history of a 'cold' that always goes to the chest. Frequently one parent has a similar history, and there may also be a family history of recurrent bronchitis and/or allergy. Allergy to house dust mites is often seen in a child from approximately two years of age who coughs repeatedly during the night and may wake in the morning coughing, sneezing and/or very congested.

 ### How is asthma treated?

Most asthma is mild and can be controlled by medication. The aims are to dilate the narrowed airways and decrease their inflammation. 'Bronchodilators' (airway openers) such as salbutamol may be inhaled from an inhaler or through a spacer (a small device that allows a younger child to breath the medicine in more easily). Bronchodilators are usually given after wheezing starts, but if they are taken before exercise they may prevent wheezing.

Preventer drugs such as cromoglycate or inhaled steroids are given by inhalation, but must be taken regularly to be effective. They are intended to prevent asthma attacks. After inhaling steroids, the mouth should be rinsed.

Oral steroids may be helpful during an acute attack, but they have to be used with caution.

If allergy to house dust mites is identified as a factor, a key part of managing and controlling the symptoms is using dust mite barrier bedding. The asthma symptoms can be significantly reduced.

Aggressive treatment is the key to controlling asthma. It's extremely important that you understand the triggers to your child's disease, and follow medication instructions carefully.

It is important to ensure that the child's environment is as free from asthma triggers as possible, e.g. using dust mite barrier bedding covers on the mattress, pillows and duvet. Other measures which can help to prevent the development of asthma in children from an allergic family or at least help to reduce the severity of symptoms include:

- not putting infants on sheepskin rugs,

- reducing clutter in the infant's room,

- reducing the number of soft toys and freezing soft toys to kill and get rid of dust mite allergens,

- using a vacuum cleaner with a micro-filter,

- not allowing pets in the infant's room.

Bronchiolitis

Bronchiolitis is a common disease of infancy and is responsible for many admissions to hospital. It occurs in children under two years of age, and usually under six months old. Respiratory syncytial virus is the most common cause, but most infants with respiratory syncytial virus will not develop bronchiolitis. Most cases occur in winter and spring. Usually the child has a mild cold for a few days, and then develops more coughing and has trouble breathing; as he or she breathes out, a wheeze or whistle may be heard. The child breathes more quickly than normal, and the lower ribs are pulled inwards with each breath. There may also be a fever. An infant with bronchiolitis may have difficulty with breast or bottle feeding especially if they are breathing fast.

 Does a child with bronchiolitis have to go to hospital?

If the child isn't too distressed, and is feeding well he or she should not need to go to hospital. More distressed infants are admitted to hospital and may receive intravenous or nasogastric fluids as well as oxygen. Antibiotics are of no value in a routine case of bronchiolitis. A chest X-ray may be done to be sure there's no secondary infection such as pneumonia. Bronchiolitis takes 7 to 10 days to resolve, but a small percentage of children have recurrent episodes; this suggests the child is asthmatic, especially if there's a family history of asthma.

Chickenpox

Chickenpox (varicella) is a very contagious viral infection; over 90 percent of the population has been infected with it. It occurs most frequently in late winter or early spring.

The infection is spread by close contact with an infected person. The illness usually appears 14 to 16 days after exposure, but the interval may be as short as 10 days or as long as 21 days. Chickenpox is infectious from 24 hours before the rash appears, until the spots have crusted over (generally 5 to 7 days).

In children, chickenpox usually begins with a low fever, followed by the appearance of a rash. The rash starts off as small, raised red bumps that later become little fluid-filled blisters. The blisters then form dry brown crusts, which fall off. Repeated groups of these sores form over the next few days. The rash most often starts on the trunk and face and spreads to the rest of the body. It may affect the mouth, eyelids, and genital area. Chickenpox is very itchy, but the illness is usually mild in children. The diagnosis is usually obvious from the rash.

 Can chickenpox lead to more serious problems?
The most common complication is bacterial infection of one or more spots. The area appears red, swollen, and painful, and antibiotic treatment may be needed. Other complications (such as pneumonia and encephalitis) are rare, and happen mainly in adults, especially those with immune-system problems. The chickenpox virus stays in the body after the rash has cleared, but is not infectious to others. Occasionally it is reactivated and causes shingles (zoster), which usually looks like groups of little blisters in one area of the body. This condition is not serious but can be persistent and very painful.

 Isn't chickenpox dangerous to an unborn child?
Chickenpox in the first 20 weeks of pregnancy may result in severe damage to the fetus, but that occurs in fewer than three percent of pregnan-

cies complicated by chickenpox. In addition, if a woman gets chickenpox a few days before or after delivering a baby, the baby may become seriously ill, because he or she has not yet developed a strong immune system. Any pregnant woman who is exposed to chickenpox and has not had the illness before (or isn't sure she has) should seek medical attention as soon as possible.

Since chickenpox is a viral illness, antibiotics aren't useful unless the spots become infected. Antiviral medication is available but isn't usually prescribed for normal, healthy children. Antihistamines, calamine, or other lotions may help prevent itching and scratching. People of all ages who have decreased immunity, as well as adults and adolescents who are exposed to chickenpox, should contact their doctor as soon as possible, since preventive treatment may be indicated. A vaccine for chickenpox has recently become available and can be purchased for use in New Zealand adults and children (Varilix).

What do I do if my child has chickenpox?

Current recommendations are to keep the child out of school or daycare until all the spots have crusted over, or for six days after the rash begins (whichever comes first).

Colds
....

'Common colds,' or upper-respiratory infections, are the most common acute infections in children. Infants and preschool children average 6 to 10 episodes a year, while schoolchildren and adolescents average 3 to 5. Children who attend daycare or live in crowded homes get even more colds. Since colds are spread by large droplets, often transferred from nose to hand, hand-washing is the most effective way to avoid spreading them.

Colds aren't serious in themselves, but can lead to complications such as ear infections and pneumonia. A fever at the beginning of a cold is normal, but a fever developing several days later suggests a secondary infection.

How can I treat a cold?

Since colds are caused by viruses, antibiotics are of no use in treating them. They are also of no value in preventing secondary bacterial infections. Bed rest is of no benefit if the child feels well enough to be up and active. Paracetamol can be given for the aches, and irritability that may accompany fever. Infants may have difficulty feeding if their noses are blocked, since they normally breathe through their noses. Small babies with stuffed-up noses may benefit from saline drops before feedings, but antihistamine–decongestant and other over-the-counter combinations have not been shown to be helpful. There is no truth to the notion that milk and dairy products increase the congestion or nasal secretions. Moreover, it's important that a child with a fever have plenty of fluids, to avoid dehydration. You may have to supply drinks often, in small amounts, if the child is reluctant to drink. Humidifiers may provide some relief from nasal stuffiness, but only a small amount of humidity is necessary as most of the moisture is deposited in the nose. Steam should be avoided because of the risk of burns.

Croup

Croup (acute laryngotracheobronchitis) is an acute but usually brief viral illness of the upper airway. It usually occurs between the ages of six months and three years, particularly around two years, and is most common in the late autumn and winter. Typically the child has a mild cold for a few days, or awakens suddenly at night with a harsh barky cough and a hoarse voice. There is a low fever, and the child may make a harsh noise when breathing in. The child is frequently upset and crying. Cough medicine will not relieve the cough.

What can I do about croup?

It may help to take the child into the bathroom and turn on the shower so the room becomes full of moisture; you can sit there and read the child a story, which is reassuring and comforting. The majority of children with croup are treated at home and do not require hospitalisation.

A child who still has difficult breathing (not just noisy breathing) should be taken to the hospital. Treatment there may consist of steroid medicine to decrease inflammation. This is usually given orally but may be inhaled or intravenous. Oxygen may also be given.

Diphtheria

Diphtheria is an acute bacterial infection that may result only in symptoms similar to those of the common cold, or may totally obstruct the upper airway, resulting in suffocation. The bacteria produce a poisonous compound (toxin) that can attack the heart muscle, cause paralysis, or even lead to kidney failure. Fortunately, immunisation has made this disease extremely rare.

Symptoms include fever, rapid pulse, swollen neck glands, and sometimes a thick yellow discharge from the nose, but the most distinctive indication is a greyish membrane on the throat and tonsils. Treatment requires hospitalisation.

Epiglottitis, see Haemophilus Influenzae B

Erythema Infectiosum, see Fifth Disease

Fifth Disease

Fifth disease (erythema infectiosum) is caused by a virus and most commonly affects school-age children, often in late winter or spring. It's spread by close contact, and symptoms begin to appear 4 to 14 days later – usually mild fever and sore throat, followed by a rash. The rash on the face is bright red and mainly on the cheeks, giving a characteristic 'slapped face' appearance. A lacy rash may be seen on the arms, legs, and trunk, and may come and go over a few weeks. The disease is most contagious before the rash appears. Joint pain is unusual in children but is quite common in women. The infection can also cause a rash without fever, or a mild coldlike illness with no rash.

Diagnosis is made by a physical examination, but may be difficult if the typical symptoms aren't present. Because it's generally such a mild illness, routine blood tests are not necessary.

 Can fifth disease cause complications?

In normal, healthy children, complications are extremely rare, but children with immune deficiency or blood diseases such as sickle cell anaemia are at risk of developing very severe anaemia. If a woman is infected with the virus during the first half of pregnancy, the fetus may become very anaemic, and may even die. Fewer than 10 percent of infected fetuses become anaemic; the reason why only some babies are affected is not well understood. During the second half of pregnancy, the risk to the fetus is almost non-existent. The virus does not cause birth defects.

 What do I do for a child with fifth disease?

There is no treatment for the disease, but children or fetuses with anaemia

 156

may require blood transfusions. Children can attend school or daycare, since they are no longer infectious once the rash appears. It's very difficult for pregnant women to avoid exposure, since the disease may be difficult to diagnose, and is infectious before the rash shows up. However, the overall risk to the pregnancy is low. Blood tests are available if a woman suspects she's been infected or exposed. If she has been infected, the pregnancy should be closely monitored.

Pregnant women, and children with immune or blood diseases, should seek medical attention if they may have been infected with or exposed to fifth disease.

German Measles, see Rubella

Haemophilus Influenzae B

Haemophilus influenzae B (epiglottitis) is an infection of the upper airway causing inflammation of the epiglottis, the flap that covers the upper airway when we swallow. It's due to a bacteria called Haemophilus influenzae B. The frequency of this disease has decreased significantly since the introduction of vaccination against this bacteria. The child, usually over three, awakens with difficulty breathing in, and appears ill and is frightened. Swallowing is also difficult, and as the disease progresses the child may drool as even saliva is hard to swallow. The child tends to sit upright and fights for every breath. In addition to the danger of a totally blocked airway, children with H. influenzae B may develop meningitis (brain inflammation). Although H. influenzae B is now a rare disease, thanks to immunisation that is almost 100 percent effective, it's a medical emergency and the child must be rushed to hospital.

Hepatitis

Hepatitis is a liver infection caused by several viruses and showing up in several forms. Symptoms may (or may not) include jaundice (yellowing of the skin and eyes), weakness, loss of appetite, brownish urine, whitish stools, nausea, discomfort in the abdomen, and fever.

Hepatitis A is highly contagious, and is spread by contamination from blood or stool. The only treatment is bed rest. Most people recover fully, and have immunity thereafter.

Hepatitis B may be more serious. Some people ('carriers') have no symptoms at all, but can infect others. A few people develop 'fulminant' (acute) hepatitis and can die of liver failure; others get a simmering chronic infection that can ultimately lead to cirrhosis of the liver or liver cancer.

 Who gets hepatitis B?

Hepatitis B is spread by body fluids, often through sexual contact or illicit drug use. It can also be transmitted from mothers to babies at birth. Mild cases are treated with bed rest and a special diet, but severe cases may require complex treatment in hospital. The best treatment is prevention; immunisation produces immunity in 95 percent of healthy children.

Lockjaw, see Tetanus

Measles

Measles is a viral infection that is preventable by immunisation. In recent years, outbreaks have occurred among preschool children as well as high-school students and young adults.

Measles is spread by personal contact and shows up after 8 to 12 days. The first symptoms are high fever, runny nose, cough, and red eyes. After three or four days, small, painless white spots appear in the mouth. A reddish rash starts on the scalp, hairline, and neck, and spreads downwards. After a few days, the rash fades and disappears, sometimes with fine peeling of the skin. Affected children usually look sick and are quite miserable. They are contagious from 3 to 5 days before the rash appears, until four days later.

Diagnosis can be made based on an examination of the child. Public-health authorities should be informed by the doctor so that they can try to prevent the disease's spread, since measles can be a severe illness.

 Does measles lead to complications?

Complications are most likely to occur in younger children, and include ear infections, pneumonia, croup, and diarrhoea. More serious complications are rare, although very occasionally encephalitis (brain inflammation) follows measles. Life-threatening complications are more common in children with immune problems.

What do I do if my child has measles?

No specific treatment has been shown to be effective for children who are not malnourished. (In developing countries, where malnutrition is a major problem, vitamin A injections are useful.) The child should not go to school or daycare for four days after the rash starts (children usually feel too sick anyway). If a bacterial infection such as an ear infection or pneumonia develops, antibiotics should be prescribed. Immunisation of people who were in contact with the child may be recommended. People who think they have measles or may have been exposed to somebody with measles should contact their doctors as soon as possible.

Mumps
· · · · · · · · · · · ·

Mumps is a viral illness, preventable through immunisation, that tends to occur in school-age children, especially in late winter and early spring. It's spread by coughing, sneezing, and talking, and shows up about two weeks after exposure. Many youngsters show no obvious sign of infection, but others develop swollen cheeks from infected saliva glands; there may also be headache, fever, diarrhoea, and irritability. The mouth may feel dry, and eating and talking may hurt. The disease is infectious from about a day before symptoms appear until about three days after the swelling goes down.

Like many viral infections, the disease is more severe in older children and adults. Painfully inflamed testicles (orchitis) occur in about a quarter of boys past puberty. Luckily, sterility is rare, but loud complaint is not! In girls past puberty, the ovaries may be involved. Viral meningitis and encephalitis are relatively common following mumps, but they tend to be mild, with severe long-term consequences being rare.

What can I do for a child with mumps?

There is no specific treatment, but soft foods and lots of fluids will help prevent mouth discomfort. Frequent toothbrushing and use of mouthwash may prevent gingivitis (gum inflammation). An icepack wrapped in a towel may relieve the soreness of the swollen glands.

Pertussis
· · · · · · · · · · · · · ·

Pertussis (whooping cough) is a highly contagious bacterial disease that begins like a normal cough but develops, after about 14 days, into a series of repetitive coughs, as the air passages become clogged with mucus. The child may turn red, or even blue, before finally taking in a long breath, perhaps with a crowing noise; this is the 'whoop' that gives the disease its popular name. Young infants are less likely to 'whoop'. Following the spasms, the child has watery eyes, and mucus streaming from the nose, and may vomit. The cough may last for several weeks.

Unfortunately, whenever the child has a cold over the following few months the cough may return, although for a shorter time. Frequently one of the adults in the house is a 'reservoir' of this infection, which then spreads to the children.

 How serious is pertussis?

The most severe cases are in younger infants, especially those under six months. The frequency and severity of pertussis have decreased since the introduction of vaccination. In New Zealand epidemics occur every 4 to 5 years. Antibiotics don't cure this disease; it must run its natural course. Untreated pertussis is contagious for three weeks from the start of the cough, but a course of erythromycin will eradicate the bacteria and shorten the infectious period. Most children should receive this drug to make them non-contagious, although it won't affect their illness. Although older children and adults eventually recover, pertussis can persist for a long time; the Chinese call it 'the hundred-day cough.' If the cough begins in the autumn, it frequently persists, on and off, until spring.

 What can I do for a child with pertussis?

Don't give cough medications, as the coughing is necessary to clear the airway. If the coughing causes vomiting, try giving smaller, more frequent meals (but not right after a coughing bout). An older child with pertussis may be more comfortable sitting up and leaning forward during coughing spasms.

 Can pertussis have serious complications?

Very occasionally, the disease leads to secondary pneumonia, seizures, or coma. In young infants the lack of oxygen during a coughing spell may rarely cause brain damage. A baby with a very severe cough may need hospitalisation so that oxygen can be supplied. If a child is turning blue during coughing spells, get medical help at once.

Pneumonia

Pneumonia is an infection in the lungs. It may be caused by many bacteria and viruses, or may be due to recurrent vomiting, or aspiration (breathing stomach contents into the lungs). Commonly the child has a mild cold for a few days before the lung infection sets in. Symptoms include fever, rapid breathing, coughing, and increasing illness. As the disease progresses, the child may develop grunting breathing and the lower ribs may be sucked in during inhalation. The younger the child, the sicker and more distressed he or she is likely to be. A doctor may be able to hear sounds in the child's chest that suggest pneumonia, but in a crying infant these are easily missed. A young infant who is ill, with difficult, rapid breathing and sucked-in ribs, may not be difficult to diagnose, but an older child with no more than a cough, low temperature, and mild illness may have a viral pneumonia that can be diagnosed only by a chest X-ray. Even then, the X-ray can't identify the type of pneumonia. Sometimes a second X-ray is done after the end of therapy, to be sure the disease has resolved.

What treatment is there for pneumonia?

The majority of children (other than infants) do not need to be hospitalised; they improve rapidly and recover totally. Although most cases are viral, it's hard to distinguish viral pneumonia from bacterial pneumonia, so an antibiotic (usually amoxicillin) is given on the chance that it will help. A particular type of pneumonia due to an organism called 'mycoplasma pneumonia' is common in older children, and especially teenagers; it responds to erythromycin. Cough suppressants have not been shown to be valuable in treating the cough that comes with pneumonia.

Does pneumonia tend to come back?

Recurrent pneumonia is uncommon in children, and when it occurs there may be some underlying cause. It's important to establish whether the child is generally well or seems to have a chronic disease. If the child is well, recurrent pneumonia may suggest asthma, especially if it's associated with wheezing. If the child isn't gaining weight, it may suggest cystic fibrosis. If the child is neurologically handicapped, it may suggest recurrent aspiration. If one area of the lung is affected repeatedly – and especially if the pneumonia is associated with some lung collapse – the possibility of a foreign body (such as a peanut) must be considered.

Roseola
•••••••••••

Roseola is caused by a virus called 'human herpes virus-6.' It occurs most commonly in children aged six months to two years, and is rare in children over the age of four. Infections occur throughout the year. It's believed that children are usually infected by family members or caregivers who have the virus but aren't ill. The disease shows up about nine days after exposure. Children are probably infectious before the rash appears.

The child develops a very high fever, with no other symptoms until the fever goes down a few days later and a fine pink or reddish rash starts on the body and spreads to the neck, arms, and legs. It lasts hours to days. Occasionally there is some stomach upset or a runny nose. Often the child is irritable while the fever peaks but playful and lively at other times.

The diagnosis is made by examining and following the child. Frequently, the cause of the fever becomes obvious only when the rash appears. Blood tests are not necessary.

Are there complications to roseola?

The most common complication is seizures that may occur at the time of the fever (see Chapter 5, 'Fever'). Roseola may occur more than once; the virus probably remains in the body and is then reactivated.

What can I do for a child with roseola?

No specific treatment is available. Any young child with a high fever (with or without seizures) should be seen by a doctor, to ensure that no more serious illness is the cause. There is no need to isolate the child.

Rubella
•••••••••••

Rubella (German measles) is a viral infection that most often occurs in late winter and early spring. It spreads directly from person to person and shows up 14 to 21 days after exposure.

In children, rubella is usually a very mild disease. The rash, usually the first sign that the child is ill, appears on the face and hairline, and later spreads to the rest of the body. Initially it consists of fine, pale pink spots, which may join up as the rash spreads. It lasts about three days. The child may have a low fever and swollen lymph glands. Joint pain is unusual in children; it's not uncommon in adolescents and adults, especially females.

Rubella can be difficult to diagnose, especially since the rash is similar to those caused by many other viral infections. Blood tests are seldom necessary, except when a pregnant woman may have been exposed or infected.

Complications of rubella in the patient are extremely rare. However, if a pregnant woman becomes infected, the baby may be severely affected by problems such as diminished birth weight, mental retardation, deafness, cataracts, heart defects, damaged retinas, and later complications such as diabetes mellitus and thyroid disease. In order to prevent exposure during pregnancy, immunisation of children is essential. Any pregnant woman who thinks she has been exposed to or infected with rubella should seek medical attention as soon as possible.

What can I do for a child with rubella?

No treatment is available for rubella. Children should be kept away from school or daycare for seven days after the rash starts.

Scarlet Fever

Scarlet fever is a bacterial infection. It's the same illness as strep throat, but with a skin rash. It's most common in school-age children, but can affect any age group. Both scarlet fever and strep throat occur throughout the year but are more frequent in the late autumn, winter, and early spring. They are spread by infected individuals, and symptoms usually appear 2 to 5 days after exposure.

Symptoms include fever, headache, vomiting, and sore throat, and the child usually feels unwell. The mouth appears very red, and the tongue is initially covered with a thick white layer. After a couple of days, the tongue looks red and swollen ('strawberry tongue'). The lymph glands in the neck may be swollen and painful. In scarlet fever, a fine pink or red rash that feels like sandpaper appears in the first 12 to 48 hours and then spreads all over the body. The rash fades within four or five days, and the skin often peels, especially on the hands and feet.

If you think your child has scarlet fever or strep throat, consult your doctor. The diagnosis can be made by examining the child. A throat culture is useful to confirm a strep infection.

Are there complications to scarlet fever or strep throat?

Complications include ear infections, sinusitis, and pneumonia. A serious but uncommon complication is rheumatic fever, a disease that may occur a few weeks after the infection and can result in permanent heart damage. Antibiotic treatment of strep infections prevents this complication. Penicillin is highly effective, but other antibiotics are available for children who are allergic to penicillin. Although the child often feels much better within a couple of days, it is very important to complete the full course of antibiotics to prevent rheumatic fever. About 15 percent of children relapse and need a second course of antibiotics.

The child is no longer infectious after being treated with antibiotics for 24 hours. He or she can then go back to daycare or school, if well enough.

Strep Throat, see Scarlet Fever

Tetanus

Tetanus (lockjaw) is caused by a potent toxin produced by bacteria. It's usually contracted in a deep wound or puncture (such wounds are often not cleaned thoroughly). The risk is greater if the wound is from something dirty, such as a nail in a garden or farmyard.

The toxin attacks the nerves in the spinal cord, producing pain and muscle spasm at the site of the wound or more generally. It can tighten the facial muscles into a fixed grin – hence its popular name. There may be fever, paralysis, and asphyxiation. The disease is often fatal. In New Zealand there were 86 cases of tetanus between 1980–1992 (mostly adults over 40 years) with eight deaths.

Immunisation is very effective in providing long-lasting protection. Booster shots are required throughout life. Be sure your family's shots are up to date, and carry a record of the shots with you; if someone has a wound away from home, the attending doctor will want to be sure the patient's immunisation is current. If a child has a deep or unclean wound, seek medical help at once.

Upper-Respiratory Infections, see Colds

Varicella, see Chickenpox

Whooping Cough, see Pertussis

CHAPTER 15

Behavioural and Learning Problems

All children display a wide variety of behaviours that concern or upset their parents at some time or other. One study showed that eight percent of preschool children in England were judged to have a 'behaviour problem' by health professionals and parents. Another study in middle-class American families showed that 18 percent of children up to five years of age were diagnosed as having behavioural disturbances severe enough to warrant intervention. A longitudinal study from Dunedin showed that nine percent of seven year old children had a stable behaviour problem. These included problems such as bedtime resistance, food refusal, resistance to toilet-training, temper tantrums, aggression, shyness, hyperactivity, and undesirable habits such as thumb sucking. Individual behavioural symptoms are very common in young children, but whether they are labelled 'problems' depends on the type, frequency, duration, and severity of the behaviour. The full range of childhood behavioural problems is beyond the scope of this book; our focus will be on problems such as shyness, aggressiveness, conduct and oppositional–defiant disorders, and attention-deficit disorder, as well as learning disabilities, which are often associated with some of these disorders.

Shyness and Aggressiveness

The way a child reacts to unfamiliar situations is strongly affected by his or her inborn temperament or personality. After the age of two, when children start to interact with other children, it becomes easier to see a trend towards shyness or aggressiveness. Neither should be considered a problem unless it clearly and repeatedly interferes in the child's life and prevents effective problem solving. It's unlikely that any major problem will result from a child's inherent shyness or aggression before the age of six years. With preschoolers one can intervene by giving a shy child a small push, or gently restraining an aggressive child. However, some very aggressive preschoolers will require professional help.

After the age of six, a child's shyness or aggressiveness can be more of a problem. Conduct and oppositional–defiant disorders are two forms of disruptive behaviour that appear in middle childhood and adolescence. At this age antisocial behaviour may be accompanied by some of the features of attention-deficit disorder with hyperactivity – including overactivity, short attention span, and lack of concentration. You can't expect to change your child's fundamental predisposition to shyness or aggressiveness, but you may be able to change the way he or she handles difficult situations.

 How do I know if my child is shy?

Shy children often avoid others, and are usually timid, easily frightened, bashful, reserved, and hesitant to commit themselves. In social situations they are often silent, speak softly, and don't take the initiative. A shy child under the age of six may regularly be bossed about by other children, or may cling to parents, fail to make eye contact, or refuse to come downstairs or into the room when people visit. However, periods of shyness are normal at five or six months of age and again at two years. If any of the following symptoms lasts more than two months, the child may be exceedingly shy:

- repeated refusal to participate with peers;

- repeated incidents of being victimised by other children;

- preference for being left alone;

- excessive clinging to parents;

- persistent fearfulness or depression.

The shyness should be considered a problem if the symptoms persist.

 What makes some children shy?

Many children appear to be shy almost from birth, and this 'constitutional' shyness may continue for the rest of their lives. Others feel shy about physical differences, and may avoid situations in which they are made to feel uncomfortable.

Shy parents often produce shy children; in other words, a tendency to shyness may be inherited. Shyness may also develop in children who are overprotected by their parents or, conversely, overly criticised by them. Children who are frequently threatened with punishment may react with fear and timidity. Those who are often teased by parents or siblings may become shy and shun social contact to avoid ridicule.

Low self-esteem can also be a factor. Children who feel insecure lack self-confidence. They are preoccupied with feeling safe and not getting hurt, and therefore don't develop social skills.

What can I do to overcome my child's shyness?

You can start by setting an example of outgoing behaviour. Let your child see you standing up for your rights when necessary, taking social risks, or seizing the initiative in difficult situations. A child who sees you starting conversations, making eye contact, and touching and staying close to people has an example to follow. Tell your child how you have overcome your shyness in various situations. For example, discuss how you introduce yourself to a stranger at a party or how you call the telephone company to complain about being overcharged.

Be careful to tackle the child's various behaviours individually. Focus attention on each situation as it happens, not on the child's overall personality. *Do not* label your child shy. Talk about the situation, without blaming the child.

Reinforce any outgoing behaviour you see in your child. Praise his or her efforts at being more independent and assertive. Point out how much you admire acts of self-confidence. For example, when your child says hello to a friend, encourage the behaviour by saying, 'You spoke to Mr. Smith very nicely. I liked the way you said, "It was nice to meet you."' Have the child's teacher help as well, rewarding behaviour such as answering questions or raising a hand to volunteer information.

Rehearsing situations that your child finds stressful is helpful. For example, go over every step of meeting a new person, including the introduction and appropriate things to say. Teach your child words and techniques for joining other children's play: 'Can I help you do that?' 'I want to play too. Which team should I join?'

As well, help your child practise ways of coping with rejection. For example, when he or she is rejected by a social clique, explain that children who know each other often stick together and don't accept newcomers easily. 'It doesn't mean that they don't like you, or that you're bad.' Remind the child of successes in previous interactions.

Many shy children feel overwhelmed in large groups, so try to provide one-on-one or small-group activities. Pair shy children with younger playmates, who are less threatening. Organise special activities in which each child takes a turn, or provide large objects that require co-operation, such as see-saws.

If you realise your child is likely to be shy in a certain situation, try subtly to make it less threatening. Arrange an entrance into the event at a good time, and let the child acclimatise before you leave. Try to smooth the path but avoid either forcing or coddling. Pushing a child into a situation doesn't teach the child how to be outgoing, and a child who is ridiculed or ignored will feel rejected.

The Aggressive Child

Aggression can be defined as behaviour that results in personal injury – psychological or physical – to someone else. For example, an aggressive child under the age of six may boss, tease, or hit other children and make them cry, or disturb everyone at a family gathering by demanding constant attention. Aggression is often triggered when a child wants something that another child has. Some preschool children even attack their parents over conflicts about feeding, bedtime, or the denial of something the child wants. There may be frequent temper tantrums. The child tends to be impulsive, immature, action-oriented, and inarticulate about feelings. Over aggressiveness is present in about one percent of 10-year-olds. Significantly aggressive behaviour is classed as a conduct disorder (see below).

What makes a child aggressive?

Some experts believe that aggression is an inborn temperament, while others feel that young children learn aggressive habits by following examples set by parents, siblings, and peers. Faulty child-rearing practices, such as a combination of lax discipline and hostile attitudes in parents, can produce aggressive and poorly controlled children. Competition, exposure to TV violence, marital strife, and fathers absent from home for extended periods are other factors believed to foster aggression.

What can I do about an aggressive child?

The most direct way to encourage your child to get along with others is to praise him or her for doing so. Use a reward system, such as a star chart or tokens that can be traded in later for actual rewards. While rewarding good behaviour and self-control, ignore aggressive acts that don't pose a threat to the physical safety of others; by paying attention to fighting or teasing, you may inadvertently reinforce this behaviour. While ignoring the aggression, do give a great deal of attention to the *injured* party, showing your concern and empathy.

When you have to correct your child's aggression, direct your remarks at the situation, not the child in general. Children become angry and resentful if they feel they're being attacked.

Remember that children are influenced by the respect you display for the rights and feelings of others. If, for example, their parents argue and belittle each other, the children will likely relate in a similar manner.

How can I prevent aggressive episodes?

Teach your child that other people's rights and needs must be respected. A good time to do this is shortly after the child has ignored or violated someone else's rights; apart from direct discussion, one approach is through role-playing. Also, teach your child to 'talk it out' rather than 'fight it out.' Give the child a list of things to do besides hitting when he or she feels upset, such as saying, 'I'm not playing any more' and leaving the group.

Aggressive children often act before they think, so if you know your child tends to be aggressive in certain situations, take a few moments to discuss how you would like things to go. Teach the child to use aggression-inhibiting sentences when angry, such as 'Count to ten' or 'Talk, don't hit.'

When your child abuses another child's rights, step in and correct the situation. Point out what's fair, gain everyone's commitment to fair play, and then withdraw. Try not to be punitive, but do get involved when a situation seems to be getting out of hand.

Can television make children more aggressive?

Many studies have shown that television has an influence on the put-downs and aggressive behaviour children use with each other. One study showed that heavy viewers of TV, especially action adventures and cartoons, were more aggressive and less co-operative with their playmates. After watching even a brief episode of TV violence, children may 'act out' in more aggressive or hurtful ways. Be aware of what your child watches – and be prepared to say no.

169

How should I punish aggression?

With younger children, a very effective form of punishment is 'time out,' in which the child is isolated – sent to his or her room, or sat on a chair – for a specified period of time. Time out is an effective way of stopping bad behaviour because it means the child doesn't receive any reinforcement (such as verbal attention or physical contact) or get any benefits from the inappropriate behaviour during the interval. If time out isn't feasible, take away privileges or have the child apologise to the injured party. Physical punishment should be avoided, since it often generates hostility and humiliation in the child. Moreover, it sets an example of aggression at the very time you are trying to teach the child to be non-aggressive.

Conduct Disorders

Many young children are disobedient and at times destructive. In preschool children, conduct problems usually show up as aggressive behaviour. In middle childhood, aggressive behaviour is still the most common form of antisocial activity but there may also be episodes of stealing, lying, and firesetting. In adolescence, antisocial activity takes the form of physical aggression, breaking into property and stealing, truancy, drug use, and sexual offences. In the normal child any such behaviours are isolated, short-lived, and mild, and tend to decrease in frequency as the child grows older. In children with conduct disorders, the behaviour occurs with greater severity, frequency, and pervasiveness over a variety of settings. The terms 'conduct disorder' and 'antisocial behaviour' are often used synonymously.

 How common are conduct disorders?

They are the most prevalent psychopathologic condition of childhood. In a survey of children aged 10 and 11 in Britain's Isle of Wight, conduct disorders were diagnosed in six percent of the boys and 1.6 percent of the girls. In Canada, about five percent of boys and two percent of girls were rated by teachers as showing conduct disorders.

 How serious are these disorders?

Children and adolescents with conduct disorders have a higher rate of depression, as well as learning and attentional problems, than other children. They often have specific learning disabilities, particularly reading disorders. (However, most children with learning disabilities do not have conduct dis-

How to recognise conduct disorders

A conduct disorder is a negative and persistent pattern of behaviour in which the basic rights of others, or the norms or rules appropriate to the child's age, are violated. The disturbance causes significant impairment in the child's social or academic functioning. It's identified by the presence of three or more of the following in the past 12 months, and at least one in the past six months:

Aggression to people and animals

● often bullies, threatens, or intimidates others

● often initiates physical fights

● has used a weapon that can cause serious physical harm to others (such as a bat, brick, knife, or gun)

● has been physically cruel to people

● has been physically cruel to animals

● has stolen while confronting a victim (e.g., mugging, purse snatching)

● has forced someone into sexual activity

Destruction of property

● has deliberately engaged in fire-setting

● has deliberately destroyed someone else's property (other than by fire-setting)

Deceitfulness or theft

● has broken into someone else's house, building, or car

● often lies to obtain goods or favours or to avoid obligations

● has stolen items of non-trivial value without confronting the victim (including forgery and shoplifting)

Serious absences

● often stays out at night against parents' instructions, beginning before age thirteen

● has run away from home overnight at least twice (or once without returning) while living in the parental home, or an equivalent

● has often been truant from school, beginning before age thirteen

Based on Diagnostic and Statistical Manual of Mental Disorders, 4th edition (DSM IV) of the American Psychiatric Association

orders.) In spite of having normal intelligence, some of these children have problems with language development and problem solving. Note that poor school performance can lead to low self-esteem and truancy.

Up to 75 percent of children with conduct disorders also have increased activity levels characteristic of attention deficit–hyperactivity disorder (ADHD). Children with both conduct disorder and ADHD tend to be even more aggressive, and to show a greater variety and severity of antisocial behaviour, than children with conduct disorders alone. Children with both disorders are at high risk of continuing their antisocial behaviour into adulthood.

 What causes conduct disorders?

The causes are the same as those of aggression in the younger child. There is strong evidence for a genetic influence; a higher than expected rate is found in the children of criminals, and if one identical twin has conduct disorders, the other has a greater than average chance of having them too. Environmental influences have also been shown to be important. Family risk factors such as marital discord and divorce, alcoholism, and psychiatric impairment are known to be associated with antisocial behaviour in children. A child whose friends show antisocial behaviour is more likely to become involved in this behaviour as well.

 What can be done about conduct disorders?

A family doctor or paediatrician may be able to counsel the family, but referral to a psychologist or psychiatrist is necessary if the behaviour is extreme, unremitting, or violent; if the child's daily functioning is significantly impaired; or if the family can't manage the child. The goal of treatment is to help the child comply with rules appropriate to his or her age, and to decrease the frequency of aggressive behaviour. With very aggressive and anti-social children it is preferable to intervene as early as possible.

One of the most effective and best-studied approaches to managing a child with a conduct disorder is training the parents to handle the behaviour, as outlined above, in the section 'The Aggressive Child.' These skills may be learned during therapy sessions and then practised at home. An alternative treatment is cognitive therapy, in which the child is taught problem-solving skills that can be used in situations that previously might have triggered aggressive behaviour. Family therapy has also been used, to establish clear communication and develop mutual negotiating skills, and sometimes family problems accompanying the conduct disorder can be treated at the same time. Also, parents may be advised to improve family relationships, channel the child's energies into positive directions, and improve the child's self-esteem. Marital counselling is sometimes indicated.

 Aren't there any medications that help?

Medication plays only a small part in the management of these children. Haloperidol has been used where aggressive outbursts take the form of frequent 'blind rages,' and Ritalin has been used for ADHD. Ritalin can also be helpful in children with conduct disorders who do not have ADHD.

Do most children outgrow these problems?

In general, children whose antisocial behaviour is limited to minor delinquent acts and who have positive relationships with other children do reasonably well. However, those who have severe antisocial problems and get on poorly with others do not. Long-term studies indicate that 75 percent of children with significant conduct disorders continue their antisocial behaviour as adolescents, and 40 to 50 percent have significant problems as adults. These problems include:

- alcoholism and drug abuse;

- increased rate of divorce, separation, and remarriage;

- criminality;

- increased school drop-out rate;

- increased unemployment;

- psychiatric problems, including neuroses and schizophrenia.

Other factors that point to problems in adulthood include conflict in the community as well as at home and in school, and any trouble involving the police.

Isn't there any way to stop this behaviour early?

It's possible that early identification of aggression and other warning signs of conduct disorder may allow these children to be successfully treated. The early signs associated with the development of conduct disorders include:

- aggressive behaviour;

- reports that the child is difficult to control;

- hyperactivity;

- oppositional behaviour (see below) after age three;

- poor relationships with siblings, including physical aggression, hostility, yelling, and teasing.

173

The more severe the disorder is at three years of age, the more likely it is to persist to eight years of age. However, if high-risk children are identified, intervention programmes may prevent future behavioural problems. These programmes should be aimed at helping the child develop social skills, self-control, and self-esteem. Parental programmes should be aimed at improving parenting skills and decreasing marital discord.

How to recognise oppositional–defiant disorder

A child is diagnosed as having the disorder only if the problem behaviour is considerably more frequent than in most people of the same mental age. The disorder has a pattern of negativistic, hostile, and defiant behaviour lasting at least six months, during which four or more of the following are present:

● often loses temper,

● often argues with adults,

● often actively defies adult requests or rules (e.g., refuses to do chores at home),

● often deliberately does things that annoy other people,

● often blames others for mistakes or misbehaviour,

● is often touchy or easily annoyed,

● is often angry and resentful,

● is often spiteful or vindictive.

Based on Diagnostic and Statistical Manual of Mental Disorders, 4th edition (DSM IV) *of the American Psychiatric Association*

Oppositional–Defiant Disorder

'Oppositional–defiant disorder' is a term often used with reference to younger children. The disorder includes negativism and hostility but, unlike conduct disorders, not the violation of societal norms. It's characterised by stubbornness, tantrums, disobedience, and defiance of authority. This behaviour reaches a peak during the 'Terrible Twos' and usually decreases afterwards, but becomes prominent again during the adolescent years.

What causes oppositional–defiant disorder?

Lax discipline by permissive parents, or unduly harsh, restrictive, or inconsistent discipline, may lead to persistent disobedience in children. Parents who are in stress or conflict, or who show little regard for the law, influence a child's readiness to obey. A very creative or strong-willed child tends to be more stubborn, and a child who is tired, ill, or hungry is less likely to obey.

What can I do about oppositional–defiant behaviour?

To prevent power struggles between you and your child, allow the child a measure of power over a situation by offering choices; for example, 'Do you want to brush your teeth before or after you wash your face?' This allows him or her to learn to solve problems, make decisions, and become more independent. Also, teach the child that when two people can't agree, a compromise allows both to give up a little and still have at least some of what they want. Try to change your position from a demand to a compromise. Use requests and suggestions rather than direct orders. A child who has advance warning, rather than being expected to obey immediately, is more likely to co-operate.

Praise your child when he or she is willing to compromise or co-operate. In addition, use a reward system, such as gold stars on a calendar or coupons to be traded in for future privileges.

Ignore minor defiance, and try to avoid head-to-head combat; instead, teach your child ways to co-operate. It's sometimes necessary to back off from a confrontation or delay a decision, when you're both upset or angry. Remember that even negative attention such as scolding can reinforce a child's misbehaviour. Threats are often difficult to carry out, and children soon learn to dismiss them.

Is there any 'best way' to make rules?

Tell your child exactly what to do and when it should be done. Instead of saying 'Clean up your room,' say 'Please pick up your toys and make your bed.' When you explain the reason for a request, the child may be more willing to comply; for example, add 'Then I'll be able to vacuum.' Make fewer rules, so they're easier to remember and enforce. State rules in a positive way: that is, tell the child what to do rather than what not to do. Say 'Please use your knife and fork' rather than 'Don't eat with your fingers.' Rules should be enforced consistently, or children will test them at every opportunity. Impose reasonable penalties if rules aren't followed, and avoid excessively harsh punishments, as well as yelling and smacking. A contract that outlines what a teen will do and what a parent will do in return may strengthen the teen's commitment to behave acceptably.

On the whole, a child is more likely to accept your discipline if you have a close relationship with abundant affection. Try to show plenty of love and caring, and spend lots of time with your child. Put up with some signs of rebellion, and let the child win some disagreements that aren't crucial, such as choices of clothes and hairstyles.

Attention Deficit–Hyperactivity Disorder

Attention deficit–hyperactivity disorder (ADHD) is characterised by inattentiveness, impulsiveness, and hyperactivity, resulting in significantly impaired functioning at home, in school, and/or with peers. In the past, various terms have been used to describe this condition, including 'minimal brain damage or dysfunction,' 'hyperkinesis,' 'hyperactivity,' and 'attention-deficit disorder.'

About 3 to 5 percent of school-age children have ADHD. It's about six times more frequent in boys than in girls. Symptoms persist into adulthood in 40 to 60 percent of people.

 Do children with ADHD always have trouble concentrating?

The symptoms may vary considerably between home and school, structured versus non-structured settings, large versus small groups, and situations with high versus low performance demands. For example, the child may have difficulty concentrating in monotonous activities but no problem in certain activities of his or her own choice, such as watching TV or playing games. Most children with ADHD have difficulty concentrating on many activities that other children enjoy, like colouring, pasting, and puzzles. They may also exhibit social immaturity and inconsistency of performance.

There is now evidence that ADHD *without* hyperactivity, also known as 'undifferentiated attention-deficit disorder (UADD),' is a separate disorder. Children with this problem function at a slower cognitive speed and appear more confused, apathetic, and lethargic, and are more likely to be depressed than children with ADHD. They also tend to be identified later, when they begin to fall behind academically in higher primary grades. Children with ADHD are described as being noisier, messier, more disruptive, less responsible, and less mature, and have more problems with peer relationships.

 Do children with ADHD have learning disabilities?

Some 25 to 30 percent of these children have a learning disability. Despite having normal, or even superior, intelligence, they are often chronic underachievers. By adolescence up to one-third have failed at least one grade in school.

Many ADHD children have language disorders, most prominent in expressive language. They may have limited vocabularies, difficulties choosing words, and poor grammar. Note that some psychologists feel language

How to recognise attention deficit–hyperactivity disorder

This problem appears before the age of seven, creates problems in at least two settings (e.g., at home *and* at school), and causes significant impairment in social or academic functioning. Also, there is impulsiveness and *either* inattention *or* hyperactivity.

Impulsiveness

- often has difficulty awaiting turn in games or group situations

- often blurts out answers to questions before they have been completed

- often interrupts or intrudes on others (e.g., butts into other children's games)

Inattention

Six or more of the following symptoms have persisted for at least six months, to a degree that is maladaptive and inconsistent with the child's level of development:

- often fails to pay close attention to details or makes careless mistakes

- often has difficulty sustaining attention in tasks or play activities

- often doesn't seem to listen when spoken to directly

- often doesn't follow through on instructions, and fails to finish schoolwork or chores (but not due to oppositional behaviour or failure to understand)

- often has difficulty organising tasks and activities

- often avoids, dislikes, or is reluctant to engage in tasks that require sustained mental effort

- often loses things necessary for tasks or activities (e.g., toys, pencils, books, assignments)

- is often easily distracted

- is often forgetful in daily activities

Hyperactivity

Six or more of the following symptoms have persisted for at least six months, to a degree that is maladaptive and inconsistent with the child's level of development:

- often fidgets or squirms in seat

- often leaves seat in classroom or other situations in which remaining seated is expected

- often runs about or climbs excessively in inappropriate situations (in adolescents this may be limited to feelings of restlessness)

- often has difficulty playing or engaging in leisure activities quietly

- often talks excessively

- is often 'on the go' or acts as if 'driven by a motor'

Based on Diagnostic and Statistical Manual of Mental Disorders, 4th edition (DSM IV) *of the American Psychiatric Association* development is linked to the development of self-control, as children use inner language to help them monitor their behaviour.

 ## Is ADHD associated with psychiatric problems?

As many as 50 to 65 percent of ADHD children have at least one additional psychiatric disorder, often including oppositional–defiant disorder or conduct disorder. Those who come from dysfunctional families with alcoholism, drug abuse, and violence are most at risk of developing serious antisocial behaviour during adolescence.

Problems with poor self-esteem are common, and 25 to 33 percent of ADHD children experience at least one episode of major depression during their childhood years. Anxiety disorders resulting in fears and worries also occur in up to 25 percent of ADHD children.

 ## What causes ADHD?

The cause is unknown, but there is evidence that the frontal lobes of the brain may be involved; they have long been known to play a critical role in regulating attention, activity, and emotional reactions. Studies have shown decreased blood flow in the frontal areas of children with ADHD. Also, PET (positive emission tomography) scans have shown that adults with ADHD have reduced brain glucose metabolism in the frontal lobes of the brain when they try to concentrate on a task. This pattern of underactivity may be due to abnormalities in the neurotransmitters (chemical messengers) in the frontal areas. It has been suggested that stimulant medication may compensate for such abnormalities, since ADHD subjects show increased activity in these frontal areas when treated with such medications.

Heredity plays a role in ADHD, since ADHD children are four times more likely to have close family members with the same problem. Also, identical twins are more likely to share ADHD than are non-identical twins or other siblings.

Birth injuries associated with foetal distress and difficult labour play a negligible role, but damage *prior* to birth may be a factor. Mothers who abuse drugs or alcohol during pregnancy have more children who suffer from ADHD and learning disabilities.

Environmental toxins, including lead, and artificial flavours, dyes, preservatives, and other food additives, have been claimed by some to be the primary cause of ADHD. Some doctors claim that sugar, food allergy, and food additives cause ADHD, and use anecdotal evidence and testimonials to back up their claims. 'Double-blind' controlled studies (in which neither the subjects nor the researchers know what substance is being administered) have shown that these are *not* important causes. It's true that recent research has shown that in a select group of children, food allergies and sensitivities to food dyes may contribute to behavioural problems and physical symptoms, although no differences were noticed in psychological test scores. Some of these studies involved preschool children with ADHD and known allergies or sensitivities, and avoidance of the triggers resulted in improved behaviour as well as fewer problems with headaches, runny noses, and sleep. But these children were not representative of ADHD children in general.

 ## How is ADHD diagnosed?

There's no single test that gives a definitive diagnosis. A history of long-standing problems of attention, impulsiveness, and hyperactivity is the best source of clues. Of course, the parents will supply one account. Because symptoms may vary with the situation, the doctor should also obtain reports from teachers concerning the child's ability to finish work, stay on task, and respect the fact that others are important. Given the association of ADHD and learning difficulties, the teachers' reports may help in assessing the level of academic achievement and general intelligence. In many cases, behavioural therapies and medication (see below) result in significant improvement in behaviour and school performance. If not, referral to other specialists may be necessary. A referral to an educational psychologist may be necessary to exclude learning disabilities. Speech and language assessment may be necessary if a communication problem is suspected. Examination of the child's emotional status may be necessary to rule out depression and anxiety disorders, and to distinguish ADHD from other disruptive behaviour problems such as conduct disorders and oppositional–defiant disorder. A medical examination is necessary to rule out visual and hearing problems, because attention and memory may be further impaired by any sensory deficits.

Various rating scales have been used to assess behaviour at home and in school. The Conners Teacher Rating Scale rates children on several aspects of behaviour, as does the Child Behaviour Check List. These scales are helpful in making an initial diagnosis and in monitoring the child's response to treatment. There are also performance tests to assess the child's ability to sustain and focus attention, as well as his or her ability to refrain from responding impulsively. These include the Matching Familiar Figures Test and the Continuous Performance Test. While these tests provide useful information, the results are not infallible, and should be interpreted in the context of all available information.

What can be done about ADHD?

The goals of therapy are to improve the child's functioning at home, in school, and with other children, through modifying his or her inattention, impulsiveness, and hyperactivity. In addition there is an attempt to improve cognitive functioning, social and behaviour skills, and self-esteem as far as possible with minimal side-effects. The long-term outcome of ADHD has been shown to improve most with a combination of parental education, medication, psychological treatments, and appropriate classroom intervention.

How do I educate myself about ADHD?

The first step is to obtain comprehensive, accurate information about ADHD, associated problems, and treatments from your doctor. Parental support groups such as the ADHD Association (PO Box 51 675, Pakuranga, Auckland) also provide important educational and support services, and give parents a forum in which to discuss problems, provide emotional support, and share effective ways to deal with schools, doctors, and service institutions.

What kinds of medication are used for ADHD?

Stimulants are commonly used, and antidepressants and clonidine (a blood-pressure medication) may also be helpful.

Stimulants such as Ritalin (methylphenidate) are the first choice. Numerous studies have shown that they are effective in more than 70 percent of ADHD children. Some 70 percent of those children who do not respond to one of these will respond to a second. Stimulants don't sedate ADHD children, but help them focus their attention, control their impulsive behaviour, and regulate their activity level. Stimulants are felt to act as neurotransmitters in certain areas of the brain, correcting a biochemical condition that interferes with attention and impulse control. Often there is a noticeable change in handwriting, talking, attention, inappropriate activity, compliance, and academic performance within just one hour of starting treatment.

Many studies have shown stimulant medications to be quite safe, and side-effects are minimal and mild. Those most commonly seen are insomnia, loss of appetite, and weight loss. Less common side-effects include sadness, depression, fearfulness, social withdrawal, sleepiness, headaches, nail biting, and stomach aches. All side-effects are short-term, and the majority disappear if the drug dosage is lowered. Long-term studies have found that children treated with stimulants do not become addicted, and the medication does not lead to illegal drug use in later years. Studies have also shown that while stimulants may cause some suppression of growth during the first year or two of treatment, this is a transient problem and the effect on adult height is minimal. Stimulant drugs are also effective in adolescents, and the dosage is the same as for older children.

For children in whom stimulants don't work and cause side effects other drugs are sometimes helpful. These include fluoxefine (Prozac), a serotonin reuptake inhibitor antidepressant, and clonidine which is a blood pressure medicine.

 ## What kind of psychological treatments are used for ADHD?

A number of psychological and behavioural therapies, alone or in combination, have been used with varying degrees of success. The aim is to modify the associated problems, such as oppositional–defiant behaviour and conduct problems.

Parental training provides a variety of management strategies for the behavioural problems seen in ADHD children. Problems such as non-compliance, defiance, and aggression are treated by the methods outlined above for the oppositional–defiant and aggressive child. This training can be offered to individuals or to groups, and involves direct instruction, modelling, role-playing, and discussion. It has been shown to be moderately effective in helping parents manage and change behaviour in ADHD children.

Family therapy deals with a variety of approaches to family-skills training, including problem solving, open and effective communication skills, anger management, and conflict resolution.

Classroom management uses procedures similar to the strategies parents learn in parental training (e.g., praise and reinforcement, and aggression management). Many well-conducted studies have proved that this improves classroom behaviour and academic performance. The ideal class for the ADHD child is highly structured and well organised, with clear expectations and a predictable schedule. The child should be seated near the teacher, and away from windows and other distractions. Because the child works slowly, he or she should be allowed extra time to complete tests and assignments. The amount of written work may be reduced until the child is better able to cope. A daily homework planner helps the child develop organisational and time-management skills. Communication between parents and teachers is important so that academic progress can be monitored.

Problem-solving training attempts to help ADHD children deal with impulsive behaviour. The children are taught to solve problems by saying to themselves, 'Stop, decide possible plans of action, do the plan, evaluate the success of the plan.' Both parents and teachers must help by modelling, promoting, and encouraging the use of problem solving. Used alone, this type of training is not as effective as stimulant therapy or behaviour-modification programmes.

Anger-management training aims to teach the child to recognise anger signals, and to use techniques like relaxation methods and coping statements to deal with the anger.

Group social-skills training is helpful for children who have poor social skills and have trouble relating to others their own age. They are taught practical techniques such as maintaining eye contact, initiating and maintaining conversation, and co-operating.

Academic intervention, in the form of individual remedial education, may be needed for children who have learning disabilities. Parents and educators work together to decide on the best classroom placement for these children. This process is generally carried out through an Individual Placement and Review Committee at the child's school.

Non-standard therapies of many kinds have been tried for ADHD and learning disorders. Although few of these treatments are harmful, most have not been proven to have any benefit. 'Orthomolecular' therapies include the use of megavitamins and essential fatty acids and various restrictive diets (allergy-free, yeast-free, sucrose-restricted, salicylate-free). 'Neurophysiologic' therapies include alpha-wave conditioning, patterning, sensory-integration training, optometric training, eye-muscle exercises, and tinted lenses. Other approaches include therapy against motion sickness, and chiropractic manipulation. None of these has been shown to be effective in double-blind controlled clinical trials.

 ## What happens when ADHD children grow up?

Long-term studies have shown that 40 to 60 percent of children who have ADHD still have symptoms in adulthood. Untreated adults are more likely to have aggressive behaviour, antisocial personality disorder, conduct disorder, depression, divorce, school drop-out, and alcohol and drug abuse. Adult ADHD is now being recognised more frequently, and treated with medications similar to those used for children.

Learning Disabilities

'Learning disabilities' (LD) is a term that refers to a varied group of disorders that show up as significant difficulties in listening, speaking, reading, spelling, writing, reasoning, and/or mathematics. These disorders are not due to environmental factors, and are presumed to be caused by dysfunction of the central nervous system. The term does *not* apply to children whose learning problems are primarily the result of visual, hearing, or motor handicaps; mental retardation; emotional disturbance; or environmental, cultural, or economic disadvantage. Most children with LD have average or above average intelligence.

What are the signs of a learning disability?

Currently, the most accepted indication of a learning disability is a significant discrepancy between a child's potential for learning and his or her achievement. Children with LD have difficulties learning in the traditional way at the accepted rate for their age group. For some reason their channels for learning don't process stimuli in the usual way. As a result, both understanding and expression can be affected. Learning disabilities affect boys and girls equally, although more boys are referred for help, perhaps because they are more disruptive to parents and teachers.

Learning problems can be divided into two main groups:

- involvement of auditory visual processes, resulting in reading disorders (dyslexia) and other language-based learning problems;

- involvement of visual and motor processes (non-verbal learning disabilities, or NLD), resulting in poor handwriting (dysgraphia), problems with mathematics (dyscalculia), and below-average social skills.

What causes dyslexia?

Dyslexia is the most common learning disability, and the one that creates the most long-term problems. It's caused not by a vision problem but by impaired language-processing skills. Dyslexics have a problem decoding 'phonemes,' the individual speech sounds in the alphabet, and have difficulty with 'phonics,' the ability to sound out words. As a result, they have trouble reading the letters of the alphabet, and so can't concentrate on the meaning of the words.

Dyslexics also have a problem with verbal short-term memory, and therefore have problems recalling letters, words, phrases, names, dates, phone numbers, addresses, and rote facts. Besides having problems with understanding written material, many of those with auditory processing problems have difficulty understanding what they hear; they may confuse words like 'dog' and 'log,' especially in a noisy environment. They may have trouble following verbal instructions.

Another problem for dyslexics is mathematics, because they have difficulty memorising basic math facts and remembering sequences of steps. They often reverse or mislabel numbers (e.g., 13 for 30), and often have difficulty understanding written math problems. Dyslexics often have a history of delayed speech, and of mispronouncing words; certain sounds are omitted, substituted, or distorted.

 ## What happens in non-verbal learning disabilities (NLDs)?

NLDs constitute about 1 to 10 percent of all learning disabilities. Problems with arithmetic and handwriting, as well as social awareness and social judgement, are associated with NLD. The right side of the brain processes non-verbal information and deals with spatial awareness, recognition of visual patterns, and coordination of visual information with motor processes (visual–motor integration). Children with NLD can have psychomotor and tactile-perceptual deficits and may be poorly co-ordinated in gross and fine motor skills. As a result, they are late learning to tie shoes, hold a pencil, catch a ball, ride a bike, and assemble puzzles. They have visual–perceptual– organisational deficits and have problems with exercises in eye–hand coordination such as handwriting, drawing, and copying from the blackboard.

In mathematics they have trouble understanding fundamental concepts, or what approach they should use to solve a problem. They may, however, have strong psycholinguistic skills such as rote verbal learning, word recognition, and spelling.

These children are often described as being isolated, with few close friends and limited social activity. They have problems understanding jokes, game strategies, the motives of others, and social conventions. They often lack insight into their own future, and their strengths and weaknesses. Possible reasons for these problems include poor social comprehension, inability to imagine the perspective of others, misinterpretation of body language, impulsiveness, and being easily led.

Are these various disorders ever combined?

ADHD occurs in 26 to 41 percent of children with learning disabilities. This combination may be due to the fact that ADHD children are inattentive and learn poorly, or 'tune out' – or perhaps some children with LD are unable to keep paying attention because the academic demands made on them are too hard, and they feel frustrated. Studies suggest that ADHD and LD are *not* genetically linked.

Depression and anxiety disorders occur in one-third of LD children, especially those with non-verbal learning disabilities. It's not surprising, since these children often have very low levels of self-esteem after years of failing at school and being labelled 'stupid' by their peers.

 What causes learning disabilities?

Heredity is a primary factor in language-based learning disabilities. As with ADHD, there is a link between learning disabilities and maternal abuse of alcohol and cocaine during pregnancy. Dyslexia is associated with dysfunction on the left side of the brain, the side specialised for language. Researchers have found that an area in the left hemisphere known as the *planum temporale*, which is normally larger on the left side than on the right, is either the same size or smaller in dyslexics.

Non-verbal learning disabilities have been found in children with severe head injuries, hydrocephalus (too much fluid within the skull), and radiation treatment of the head. Since these conditions involve destruction of white matter in the right hemisphere, it's felt that NLDs are caused by early damage to this white matter.

 How are learning disabilities diagnosed?

It's important that a diagnosis be made before skill levels and self-esteem slip to dangerous lows. The child's doctor should look for any neurological dysfunction, and assess hearing and vision to rule out sensory or neurological problems affecting learning. The doctor should also take a history of developmental milestones to rule out mental retardation and autism, and ask about behaviour and attention span. Medications such as antihistamines, anticonvulsants, tranquillisers, and asthma drugs can affect attention and learning. Formal assessment of intelligence and educational achievement, by a psychologist, is occasionally necessary. Reports from teachers and/or IQ tests can give information about the child's cognitive strengths and weaknesses, and may help define how well the child processes information. Some of the more frequently used intelligence tests for school-age children are the Wechsler Intelligence Scale for Children (WISC-III) and the Stanford-Binet Intelligence Scale. Academic achievement can be assessed by tests such as the Peabody Individual Achievement Test–Revised (PIAT–R), and the Wide Range Achievement Test–Revised (WRAT–R).

 ## What can be done about learning disabilities?

The cornerstone of treatment is educational therapy, tailored to the child's individual needs and depending on his or her learning strengths and weaknesses. There are many programmes to teach reading skills, including intensive phonetic teaching programmes.

Besides remedial reading techniques, some teachers have tried instructing LD children in learning strategies. There has been some success in teaching them to improve the way they approach new tasks, memorise new information (such as using mnemonics), and organise information (such as using rhymes or visual images to link bits of information together). One successful strategy is the 'write–say' method, in which the student rewrites incorrectly spelled words several times while spelling the words out loud. A variant of this method has proved successful in teaching multiplication tables.

Other methods of helping LD children include having other children in the class or school act as tutors, and using computer-assisted instruction. Children with writing disorders may be helped by homework buddies, oral testing, using a classmate's notes, and being taught keyboarding.

Social-skills training, psychological counselling, and behaviour-management techniques are often used, but have not been shown to be consistently helpful. In the child with LD and ADHD, stimulant medications have been shown to improve classroom performance, not only through improved attentiveness, but also in the way the central nervous system processes information. In reading tasks, this effect is seen in improved word-finding abilities.

Schools and special education services are required by law to provide specialised education for LD children. This may mean special classes, special teachers, or even a special school. There is evidence, though, that teaching LD students in regular classes, using highly motivated, well-trained teachers and teachers' aides, can lead to improvements in academic performance, behaviour, and self-esteem.

Where can I get more detailed information about LD children?

One of the most valuable supports for parents is the Parent and Family Resource Centre Inc. PO Box 9407, Newmarket, Auckland. It provides parents with information about local services and new discoveries, and offers support groups in which parents can compare notes and encourage each other. For more information on this and other groups mentioned, see 'Further Resources,' at the end of the book.

 What happens when LD children grow up?

Most children with reading disability can compensate and attain literacy, but as adults they may do less well in work as well as in social and psychological adjustment. The outcome is better for those who are of higher intelligence, have a less severe disability, are in a higher socio-economic class, attend private school, are not hyperactive, and have no known neurological problems. With the right support systems, many people with LD achieve high academic and professional success; two good examples are Winston Churchill and Thomas Edison.

CHAPTER 16

The Child with Chronic Pain

• •

There are few problems more distressing to parents than seeing their own child in pain. None of us wants to see our children suffer, and our instinctive reaction is to do our utmost to bring relief from the pain. Usually we think of pain as a sudden, acute sign of potentially serious problem that needs immediate attention: an accidental knife cut, a sprained ankle, acute appendicitis.

Not all pain is like that. 'Chronic' pains tend to occur over and over again, sometimes in predictable patterns. The problems considered here are familiar to many experienced parents, and include recurrent stomach-aches, headaches, teething pains, growing pains, and others.

Q How can I tell if my child's pain is serious?

Unlike that for acute pain, the time frame for many chronic-pain problems may be weeks, months, or even years. The child may not be obviously unwell, but may have been complaining about the same symptoms for a very long time. Parents might be ready to accept similar symptoms in themselves or another adult, but in the case of their children they worry that some major problem is being overlooked. Their fears may grow worse if they hear stories from other parents or relatives about someone's illness being missed or misdiagnosed. On occasion, parents are convinced that there must be something wrong simply because the complaints have lasted so long. In fact, the reverse is often true: the shorter the duration, the more likely it is that the pain is due to an illness or abnormality – although time alone is not a reliable way to judge the cause or seriousness of pain.

Most of the situations outlined below are common in childhood, and most can be dealt with by parents without much medical intervention.

 188

However, there are always exceptions, and each child needs to be considered individually. No written advice (not even this chapter!) can substitute for careful assessment of the child's problems. This chapter is written in the hope of helping you understand some chronic-pain scenarios – *not* as a specific aid to diagnosis.

Recurrent Abdominal Pain

'Recurrent abdominal pain' (RAP) is the name commonly used to describe the symptoms of children who complain of repeated episodes of stomachache or pain. From 5 to 10 percent of children experience RAP at one time or another. It's so frequently seen by paediatricians that it has been a subject of study in pediatric journals for decades. Each year there are new theories about the cause, and each idea rides a wave of popularity for a while. Causes suggested in both the medical and lay press in recent years include:

- *lactose intolerance* – an inability to digest the sugar commonly contained in milk and milk products, resulting in gas, cramps, and sometimes diarrhoea (see Chapter 12, 'Feeding Your Child');

- *gastroesophageal reflux* – regurgitation of acid from the stomach upwards into the oesophagus (swallowing tube), sometimes causing a sensation of pain or 'heartburn' (see Chapter 7, 'Spitting up, Vomiting, and Diarrhoea');

- *H. pylori infection* – ulceration and inflammation caused by *H. pylori*, a bacteria that lives in the stomach. While this can occur in children, and can cause pain, there are also studies showing that it can occur just as frequently in children without pain. It may be *a* cause, but it's certainly not *the* cause;

- *food allergy* – a convenient diagnosis for a wide variety of problems that don't have an easy solution. It's wise to be sceptical. If there is not a clear and obvious reaction to a specific food each time it's consumed, it's unlikely to be the culprit, no matter what the allergy tests may show (see Chapter 12).

 How can I tell what's causing my child's abdominal pain?

The vast majority of children with this problem will never be diagnosed with a 'disease' related to it. Nevertheless, there are several factors that may contribute to the situation, and you should consider all of them.

Start with the question of language. Most children don't willingly describe the pain; they usually say, 'My tummy hurts,' and *we* interpret that as a statement of pain. In fact, very young children use the expression 'hurts' to describe any sensation outside their usual range of experience. Try suggesting that the child go to the bathroom as a first step in relieving a 'tummy-ache'; the sensation that adults recognise as a need to pass a bowel movement may well be a 'hurt' to a young child. Similarly, they may say 'hurts' to describe a variety of other sensations, including nausea, nervousness or 'butterflies,' hunger, a full feeling after a meal, mild cramps, or the need to urinate. Depending on the nature of your response, this descriptive pattern may become ingrained, and may remain part of the child's vocabulary in later years.

Parents can be good detectives if they look for other clues to the significance of the pain. By using examples the child recognises, you may be able to narrow down the problem. For example, 'Does it feel like you have to throw up? Does it feel like you have to do poos or wees? Does it feel like you ate too much?' A good detective is also a good observer. Note the time pattern of recurrent pain (just before leaving for school, just before bedtime, or after meals, for example), and see how the child looks when he or she complains. Sometimes a child talks about pain in a very matter-of-fact manner, and a few minutes later goes out to play. It's particularly important to see how much the pain interferes with activities the child enjoys (playing with friends, etc.), as opposed to those he or she may not enjoy (such as school).

RAP is often associated with constipation. Sometimes the problem is evident; the child simply doesn't have a bowel movement very often. But there are also children whose constipation is less apparent; they seem to move their bowels daily, but they still have a lot of stool backed up in the bowel, causing frequent cramps. Studies have shown that many of these children get pain relief when fibre is added to their diets, even though they've never complained of constipation. Occasionally, children develop patterns of stool-withholding that may be difficult for them to change on their own. These children tend to have a large accumulation of stool in the large bowel, and may pass a bowel movement in the toilet only once every few days. The movements tend to be very large. In between, they may have 'accidents,' soiling their underwear with stool that seeps down past the accumulation in the rectum. This problem, called 'encopresis,' may also cause cramps and complaints of abdominal pain. (See Chapter 6, 'Toilet-Training.')

Events in the child's environment (home, family, and school) may also be factors in recurrent abdominal pain. Children tend to be creatures of habit, and major changes in their world can be quite disruptive. Some express their upset or anxiety in words, but others show the stress through a variety of physical symptoms, including abdominal pain. Moving, resulting in a change in city, home, and/or school, is disturbing to many children. The death of a relative, or even a pet, is difficult for them to understand and may trigger problems. The birth of a baby brother or sister is almost guaranteed to produce some degree of jealousy (in other words, it's normal), but may have a greater impact on some children. Finally, tensions within the home, especially marital difficulty, virtually always affect children to some degree.

Although it may seem hard to believe, abdominal pain can actually be rewarding to some children. Being ill usually attracts parental concern and attention, which sometimes reinforces a pattern of behaviour that may have started quite innocently. When the parents are separated, a child's illness is often the only thing that will bring the pair together around the child.

Is abdominal pain ever hereditary?

In thinking about your child's pain, also take a close look at yourself. Parents with chronic abdominal problems are more likely to have children with RAP. Some adults have intestinal symptoms on a regular basis without necessarily having a disease. Do you have irritable-bowel syndrome? Do you get diarrhoea whenever you're nervous or upset? Do you have a sensitive stomach? Do you vomit more easily than most people? Do you have problems with chronic constipation? A 'yes' to any of these questions may indicate that the pattern runs in the family. In other words, the apple doesn't usually fall far from the tree! The situation may be intensified by the fact that adults who have these problems tend to focus on them, and may talk about them in front of their children, so that the children have considerable exposure to the issues during their formative years.

You should also take a close look at your own concerns and anxiety. If a relative has recently died of stomach cancer, for example, you may be particularly worried about stomach pain in your child. While there's no reason to suppose there's any link between the two, the worry is understandable. By recognising the source of your concern, you may be able to keep it in perspective, and avoid increasing your child's anxiety. Admit your concern to the doctor; it's likely that the disease you fear can be easily ruled out.

How often is abdominal pain a sign of serious disease?

Obviously, not all recurrent abdominal pain can be attributed to the causes and circumstances above. Pediatric textbooks contain literally hundreds of causes of such pain. However, those hundreds of causes account for about five percent of all the children who have this symptom. For the remaining 95 percent, no obvious disease is found.

Understandably, no parent wants his or her child to be part of the five percent with a disease, and many parents push for tests to rule out serious illness. Unfortunately, children are frequently overtested for this reason. Testing for the sake of 'ruling out,' in the absence of any evidence to suggest a particular diagnosis, is rarely helpful. Often it does more harm than good, by inflicting procedures that make the child feel even more ill and vulnerable. It's far more valuable to spend time reviewing the issues listed above than to go on a 'fishing expedition' of laboratory tests and X-rays.

 ## What if no serious illness is found?

If your child belongs to the 95 percent whose pain can't be related to a specific disease, you should be relieved; that's usually better than the alternative. If you find this conclusion difficult to accept, and fear that something may have been overlooked, it's important that you feel comfortable enough with your doctor to ask questions until all your concerns have been answered.

Even more important, don't assume that your child is 'making up' the symptoms. Pain is a very subjective sensation, and we all learn different thresholds (tolerances) for pain as we grow up. The abdominal discomfort may be very real to the child even though no disease is involved. After all, an adult who develops diarrhoea when nervous, or who becomes nauseated at the sight of blood, isn't 'making up' these symptoms, yet they aren't related to disease. They are just examples of how closely the stomach and intestines are linked to the brain and emotions – in both adults and children.

When abdominal pain is important

There are a few circumstances that do call for prompt medical assessment. If your child's recurrent abdominal pain is associated with weight loss, recurrent fevers, chronic diarrhoea, blood in the stools, pain or difficulty with urination, or frequent vomiting, you should certainly see a doctor. The location of the pain may also be noteworthy. Usually, children point to their navels as the site of pain; if the pain is persistently on one side, or if it's felt in the back, further assessment is usually appropriate.

In the absence of specific illness, what can you do to help your child? Details depend on the situation, but here are some general tips that may be helpful.

- Don't ask about pain if the child hasn't brought the subject up, and never ask if he or she had any pain today. If you do, most children will say yes; if you don't, the child may not mention it. You can be sure that if the pain is significant, the child will refer to it. If the subject isn't discussed, the pattern is less likely to be reinforced and may ultimately disappear.

- Teach the child ways to deal with the discomfort without disrupting the rest of the household. He or she may want to go to the bathroom, and then perhaps lie down in the bedroom for a little while until the feeling passes. (Similarly, it's preferable that the child lie down for a few minutes in the school nurse's office rather than come home.)

- If psychological or social stresses may be playing a role (the death of a relative, a recent move, marital problems), they need to be dealt with openly. Professional counselling may be appropriate. Note that the focus of the counselling needn't be the abdominal pain, but rather the stresses that underlie it.

- Display an attitude of understanding and empathy, while encouraging your child to participate in normal routines as far as possible. School attendance is particularly important.

- Avoid extremes in dietary habits, and try to maintain regular mealtimes. While most recurrent abdominal pain is not due to food allergy or intolerance, some children are sensitive to excesses in their diet. For example, those who drink huge amounts of fruit juice each day, especially apple juice, may have abdominal discomfort. By the same token, adding a little fibre to the diet – in the form of whole wheat bread, popcorn, fibre cereals, or high-fibre cookies – may reduce the symptoms.

Growing Pains

It's not at all clear how 'growing pains' got their name. There's no real evidence that they have anything to do with growing, except that they seem to occur exclusively at an age when children are growing rapidly. The term refers to pains in the legs; although there's no clear explanation for them, they are indeed real. Furthermore, they have some characteristics that are common enough to be very helpful in establishing a diagnosis.

Typically, these pains occur in children between the ages of three and 10 years, particularly towards the younger end of that range. They usually come at night, often while the child is in bed, and seem to affect mainly the lower legs, especially the knees and shins. In most cases it's not difficult to distinguish growing pains from other, potentially serious problems in the legs. Here are some hints.

- Growing pains generally affect both legs. An injury or other abnormality is more likely to involve one leg, not both.

- The pain often comes when the child is motionless and not putting weight on the legs. In almost any other problem of bone, joint, or muscle, the pain is worse when the affected part is in use, or at least bearing weight.

- The child gets relief from someone rubbing or massaging the affected area. A child with a sore joint or a bruise doesn't like to have the area touched.

- Once asleep, the child rarely awakens until morning, and at that time is usually fine. More serious problems are unlikely to resolve that quickly.

- If the child limps, growing pains are very unlikely to be the cause. Consult your child's doctor.

 What can be done about growing pains?

As with most problems in childhood, there's a wide spectrum of severity. Most children have a pattern that's easily recognisable and doesn't need any investigation. A few have pain that is not typical and may be unusually bad. These children may benefit from a referral to a doctor experienced with such problems, and may require some tests before a diagnosis can be made. There is no test for typical growing pains, however. The diagnosis is made by recognising the classic pattern, and by checking that there's no evidence to suggest any other cause.

Treatment tends to be simple. A pain reliever such as paracetamol may provide relief at bedtime. (Asprin should be used with caution in children; see the remarks on Reye's syndrome in Chapter 5, 'Fever.') Massage of the area, or application of heat, may also be helpful.

Teething Pain

Does teething cause pain? It may seem like heresy even to ask such a question, since generations of parents have been absolutely convinced that it does. Teething has also been alleged to cause fever, rash, diarrhoea, and vomiting in young infants. Yet, despite the fact that teething is a universal phenomenon, there's not a shred of reliable evidence that it plays a role in any of these common childhood problems!

In many cultures, teething is seen as a disease requiring specific intervention and treatment. Is it conceivable that millions of parents, grandparents, and great-grandparents could be wrong? Let's consider some facts.

From the time they're born, newborns are continually exposed to a variety of common viruses, carried by adult caregivers and siblings who may not, themselves, be ill. The most common signs of illness when infants are infected with such viruses are fever, rash, and diarrhoea – the same signs attributed to teething. Why, then, does teething get the blame? The usual sequence of events is as follows: A parent notes that the infant is warm, has a rash, or has diarrhoea; the parent then looks in the baby's mouth, and specifically at the gums; from about 3 to 4 months of age until 2½ years of age, there is virtually *always* a tooth in the process of erupting. As soon as the parent sees the swollen gum, he or she assumes that the diagnosis has been made. But if the parent looked at the gums on a day when the baby had no symptoms, he or she would probably see a very similar picture!

 ## Surely teething must cause some pain?

It may be reasonable to assume that the little bit of swelling and redness observed over the gum just before the tooth breaks through involves slight discomfort, but there's no logical way to connect this to the other symptoms described above. Even when babies drool and put things in their mouths, it's not clear whether this is because of gum pain or is simply part of normal development. After all, some normal children don't show a tooth until 12 months of age, but they still start putting things in their mouths at 4 to 5 months.

The danger of blaming illnesses on teething is that it may prevent us from looking for the real cause. While most fevers are due to viruses that will get better on their own, without treatment, occasionally an infant develops a more dangerous infection. With very young babies it can be difficult to tell the difference between minor and major illnesses, and assessment by an experienced doctor may be very important.

 ## Since teething isn't a disease, does it require treatment?

There's no shortage of teething preparations in any drugstore, but in general it's wise to avoid them. There have been rare instances of children suffering serious side-effects when such medicines were improperly used, or when they got into the wrong hands (such as a two-year-old eating an entire tube of teething gel). While such incidents may not be likely, it hardly seems worth taking chances just to treat a 'non-disease.' After all, what could be more normal than a healthy baby growing teeth? It's just part of human growth, and we should treat it as such.

Headache

Like abdominal pain, headache tends to be a recurrent phenomenon in some children. Although many parents have the idea that children shouldn't get headaches, they are in fact quite common, especially in school-age and ado-lescent children. A headache is frequently part of a viral illness in a child, as it is with an adult; this situation can often be recognised by fever and other accompanying symptoms, such as a sore throat and swollen glands.

 Why do some children get headaches if they're not sick?

Simply put, some children are headache-prone. Often at least one of the par-ents has the same problem. The pattern of recurrent headaches may develop at a fairly young age, but is more likely to start after children are in school. The children are otherwise healthy and function normally in every way. The most common cause of the headache is migraine, which also tends to run in families.

 What happens in migraine?

Migraine is best understood as a change in the size of the blood vessels that carry blood to the brain. Arteries, being lined by muscle, have the ability to become narrow or wider. In migraine headache, the arteries first constrict

---

Headaches and brain tumours

The underlying fear of every parent whose child has headaches is that there may be an ominous problem caus-ing them, and a brain tumour is the worst fear; although parents rarely mention the possibility, they usually acknowledge having thought about it. But brain tumours are among the *rarest* causes of headaches in children. When they are the cause, they characteristically produce a pattern of early-morning headache and vomiting, and the headache itself may gradually become unrelenting. Any child whose headache is associated with early-morning vomiting, seizures, difficulty with speech or movement, or a change in consciousness should obviously be seen by a doctor as soon as possible.

(become tighter), sometimes causing symptoms such as visual disturbances or 'funny feelings,' and then dilate (become wider). When they dilate, the headache usually begins.

Children with migraine often feel nauseated, and may even vomit. They frequently like to avoid bright light and loud noises, and may be most comfortable if they lie down in a dark room and try to sleep. Migraine may be triggered by fatigue, exercise, or long periods in the sun. Also, food triggers can sometimes be identified, and it may be valuable to keep a record of what was eaten just prior to a headache, to see if a pattern emerges. Common culprits include nuts, caffeine (as in cola drinks), and spiced meats, among others. With time, both parents and children become expert in identifying the pattern of migraine. They can usually tell when an episode is beginning, and they know what to do.

What can I do for a child with migraine?

Most children with migraine can be treated with the simple measures listed above, and with paracetamol. Note that it's important to give medication as early as possible. In an effort to avoid using medicine unnecessarily, parents sometimes wait to see if the headache will disappear on its own. The longer a migraine headache has been present, the more difficult it is to get rid of. Therefore, once you are familiar with your child's migraine pattern, treat it early rather than late. Be sure that school staff also know how to proceed.

Some migraine is particularly troublesome and doesn't respond to these simple measures. If so, consultation with a doctor is strongly advised.

What else can cause headaches in children?

Tension headaches are the other major cause. While they are more common in adolescents, they can occur in preteens as well. These headaches produce a sense of tightness around the head, especially over the temples. The neck muscles may also be tight.

Typically, tension headaches are a response to stress. Most of us have experienced them at one time or another – after a particularly difficult day at work or an emotionally draining event at home. Children and teens are no different in their responses to stress; the challenge may be to find out what the stress is. Indeed, the children themselves may not recognise the stresses affecting them.

If children aren't willing to talk openly about these issues with their parents (sometimes because the home environment is part of the problem), professional help may be necessary. As a first step, the problem should be discussed with the family doctor or paediatrician. A referral to a psychologist or psychiatrist may be recommended. With such expert help it should be possible to understand the underlying issues; also, many psychologists can teach the child methods of self-relaxation to help relieve the headaches. A child who gains more control of what happens to his or her body will be less vulnerable to headaches.

Chest Pain

Chest pain is not very common in children, and it always frightens parents, probably because they have been warned to think of it as an early sign of a heart attack. In children, heart problems very seldom cause chest pain. In fact, even in children who are born with heart abnormalities, chest pain is quite rare.

How do you find the cause of a child's chest pain?

In most cases, tests are not very helpful. The story of the pain is far more useful; by asking the right questions, an experienced doctor can often decide whether or not X-rays or other tests need to be done. Even anxiety and depression can cause chest pain, and in these cases it's more important to find the cause of the problem than to provide pain medication.

The commonest cause of chest pain in children is 'musculoskeletal,' meaning that it comes from muscle or bone. The entire chest wall is lined with muscles (they help you breathe), and a cramp or spasm in one of the muscles can cause a sharp pain, especially when the child takes a deep breath. (Some people call this a 'stitch.') Some children and adolescents are particularly prone to this. Also, just as muscles in the leg can get sore or pulled from overuse, so can muscles in the chest. A child with a violent cough may eventually develop chest pain from all the strain, although this usually improves as the cough gets better.

'Heartburn,' another cause of chest pain, has nothing to do with the heart. It is essentially the same problem as gastroesophageal reflux, discussed above, under 'Abdominal Pain,' in which acid from the stomach regurgitates upwards into the chest area. This is less common in children, but does occur, and often causes a burning pain in the centre of the chest.

Don't feel you have to figure out chest pain on your own. A visit to the doctor will often sort out whether a significant problem exists. Recognise that most causes are minor and improve with time. However, any chest pain that is severe and persistent, or that causes shortness of breath, needs medical assessment.

CHAPTER 17

Research: Being Part of the Picture

T he advice in this book is based not just on the opinions of experienced doctors and nurses but on scientific research into what can be *proved* to benefit children with various problems. Because we consider careful medical and clinical research to be of great importance, we want to conclude with a few comments about what research is, and what it means to our children. This is especially important as you and your child may someday be asked to participate in a research project.

What's the difference between medical research and clinical research?

Research in the field of medicine includes a variety of approaches to collecting information. It can roughly be divided into *basic medical research* and *clinical research*. Basic medical research usually goes on in specialised laboratories, and involves attempts at understanding the underlying principles of health, diseases, and/or therapies. Patients are rarely involved in this form of research. In contrast, clinical research often involves the participation of patients, and its direct aim is to develop and test better ways of diagnosing and treating people.

What happens to patients in a research study?

In many cases, clinical research is limited to measuring or observing the course of health or illness at a given time, or over a time period. Observation may include questions (about illness symptoms, activities, past illnesses, and so on), physical measurements (such as weight and height), and/or tests (such as blood tests or X-rays).

Unfortunately, studies like these often fail to reveal whether treatments or tests actually benefit people in a significant way. For this reason another type of clinical study, called a 'randomised controlled trial,' is sometimes used. This is designed to compare two or more different approaches to treatment. Usually each of the approaches must be either an established treatment, or a new method that is believed to be as good as, or better than, the standard approach. For example, if the usual approach to an illness is to observe it without treatment, and a new drug becomes available to treat the illness, the trial might consist of one group getting observation and another getting the new drug. Both groups would then be evaluated to determine which fared better, and the most successful approach would then become standard.

 Why are these trials called 'randomised' and 'controlled'?

The groups to be compared have to be similar at the start of the trial (e.g., they should have the same range of severity of illness and be the same mix of ages). Otherwise it may not be clear whether a difference at the end is due to the treatment approach, or to the original differences between the groups. To assure that the groups start out as identical as possible, participants are assigned to the groups by a process of chance called 'randomisation.' This is similar in effect to flipping a coin – if heads are up, the person joins one group; if tails are up, it's the other group – and means that each participant has exactly the same chance of ending up in one group or the other.

The trials are often 'controlled' in other important ways. Often the participating patients don't know what treatment they're receiving. In the example above, the group getting the medication might 'feel better' just because they *believed* the pills were helping; to keep the test fair, the group not getting medication might be given a placebo (dummy drug) so that they received the same imaginary benefit. Often even the researchers don't know who's getting what, to be sure that their opinions don't affect the results; these are called 'double-blind' trials.

 Are these studies done on children too?

Clinical research, and in particular randomised controlled trials, play a very special role in improving the medical care of our children. Doctors have learned that even the most thoughtful judgements or expert opinions about how to treat an illness often have to be revised when good studies are finally performed. Also, the illnesses that affect children, and their responses to treatment, are so specific to children that experiments or studies carried out on animals or adults with similar illnesses usually don't tell us how the treatment will affect a child. If we didn't do clinical research with children as participants, we would be neglecting them. While progress was made in treating adult illness, many of the essential questions about childhood medical care would go unanswered.

Good clinical studies sometimes have a lot of rules for deciding which group a child is placed in, and who can know which treatment a child is receiving, and so on. These rules may seem restrictive, and even frustrating, to parents, but they are usually essential to make the trial reliable. Without them, the validity of the information gained in the study would be in question.

Who runs these clinical studies?

Some doctors and nurses are involved in designing and running clinical trials in their hospital departments or practices. General practitioners often play a critical role in referring patients to studies that need to recruit wide participation, and they may play a further role by following the people in the study, gathering information, and helping to ensure that patients get the tests and treatments needed. Note that if a child's doctor refers a child to a study, he or she usually *remains* the child's doctor, with the responsibility of caring for the child's health whether the child remains in the study or not.

If my child takes part in a study, will our doctor necessarily be involved too?

Your child's doctor may have very little to do with the research your child participates in. However, even if your child joined the study through another doctor or nurse, your child's usual doctor will probably appreciate hearing about it. He or she may have advice or support to offer both you and your child. No one has studied whether doctors involved in conducting research, or in referring participants to research studies, provide better care than other doctors. Many of the latter may have an interest in research but not be in a position to participate, or may not have been approached. However, doctors who actively participate may be showing a greater appreciation of the importance of research, and a greater sensitivity to the steady progress of medical knowledge and care. If you have questions about the role your child's doctor will play when your child takes part in research, it may be well worth your while to ask him or her about it.

What do I need to understand about my child taking part in research?

Most people recognise that participation should be voluntary, and that participants should understand the purpose and nature of the research they take part in. This means that no one should be forced to join a clinical study through threats, bribery, or fear of not getting treatment otherwise.

As you can imagine, these principles are less easily applied to children. Many simply can't understand the purpose and nature of the research, because they are too young or, in some cases, because of handicaps. They are therefore unable to give meaningful consent.

If people who are incapable of understanding the research are simply left out of clinical studies, the studies will not be complete; also these individuals will be denied the chance to contribute to, or perhaps even benefit from, the research. Therefore, a compromise appears to be the best solution; the parent or guardian examines the purpose and nature of the research, as well as its risks and benefits; makes the decision; and gives permission on behalf of the child if participation seems worthwhile.

Children over seven or eight years of age may be interested in participating in this decision, even if they aren't mature enough to fully understand or appreciate the study. Therefore, their opinion should be considered in addition to that of the parent or guardian. This way, children can participate in and benefit from research, but their rights as individuals are still respected.

 ### How do I find out the purpose and nature of the study?

The doctor, nurse, or research assistant who contacts you should be able to outline the key information. In addition, most studies are required to give you a letter explaining the most important aspects. When you receive it, you should be able to see clearly what question the study is designed to answer, and get a sense of whether you feel the study is worthwhile. You should also get a clear description of what the study involves. This includes how long it will run, what tests and treatments will be used (and what these tests and treatments are like), whether your child will be assigned to a particular group and treatment by randomisation, and what the alternatives to participation are. You should also be informed of your right to withdraw your child from the study at any time, for any reason.

 ### How do I balance the possible risks and benefits?

When reviewing the study information, pay special attention to the possible risks or harms as well as the benefits. An example of a very minor harm is the discomfort and bruising that occurs when a blood sample is taken from a child's vein. A more significant risk or harm might be the chance of a severe skin reaction to one of the medications being studied, if that medication is known to cause such a reaction.

Most treatment approaches, new and old, involve some degree of risk or harm. There are no easy rules for balancing these against the benefits. Yet it makes sense that, for the individual, the potential benefits should outweigh the potential harms. For example, it may be acceptable for a child to have a single blood test for research that will help other children. However, in most cases it's not acceptable to subject a child to many blood tests, or more distressing tests, for research that benefits only other children. In addition to this, the potential risks and benefits of the different approaches in a randomised controlled trial should be fairly balanced. For example, if a new medication is known to have side-effects much worse than those of the traditional medication, and if the potential benefits from the new medication are clearly small, one could argue that the treatments aren't balanced and that the study is improper.

As for the benefits, they can be divided into three categories. First, the study results may help children as a whole, or a specific group of children, through improved medical knowledge. This knowledge may not necessarily benefit your child directly, but your child gains indirectly by helping others, taking pride in this contribution, and knowing that other children continue to contribute in this way. After all, the knowledge from similar studies may have helped your child in the past, or may help in the future. Second, your child may benefit personally from the knowledge gained through the study, if, for example, it compares two medications and clearly indicates which is best. Third, your child may benefit by receiving treatment that is still being tested and is not yet generally available. The extra attention (information, observation, and so on) the child receives may also be beneficial.

Fortunately, you aren't left to balance these issues alone. When a research study is paid for by a large governmental research-funding organisation (such as the Health Research Council or by an organisation such as the National Child Health Research Foundation, it has already gone through independent, rigorous, competitive review. This review process works towards ensuring that only the best, most scientifically sound studies are selected for funding. These large organisations also require that the studies be reviewed by a special group called an 'ethics committee.' Ethics committees are usually made up of people from a variety of backgrounds, such as philosophy, medicine, and nursing, and often include members from the community (at a children's hospital, parents of children who have required medical care are often selected). These groups examine the clinical studies to be sure that the risks and benefits are reasonable, and that appropriate information is given to the parents.

What if the trial is paid for by somebody else?

When clinical studies are paid for by other organisations, such as drug companies, they may not go through quite the same process of review. Most universities and hospitals require all studies conducted on their premises, including those funded by drug companies, to be approved by the ethics committee. The Starship Children's Hospital does. Because some studies undergo extensive review and others don't, you should feel free to ask who is paying for the study, and what reviews have been done.

Even though these reviews ensure that most clinical studies are appropriate for children to participate in, you and your child have the final decision. It is also important to remember that the ethic's committees in New Zealand all require that you and your family have sufficient time to consider the research project before deciding whether or not your child will participate. You should never feel as though you are being pressured to make a quick decision. Your child's doctor may assist you with the decision, but ultimately you yourself should be satisfied that you understand the benefits and the drawbacks of any research in which your child takes part.

CHAPTER 18

Emergency First Aid

Anyone who takes care of children should understand the basics of first aid. Injuries can happen any time, and the first few minutes can be critical. Even when an injury isn't serious, prompt and appropriate first aid can make the difference between a minor incident, quickly forgotten, and a frightening and upsetting one.

This chapter gives a brief overview of what to do in a few basic emergencies; for more complete and extensive training, take a first-aid course from an agency such as the Red Cross or the St. John Ambulance Society. Even if you never have to deal with a serious situation, the training will change the way you handle day-to-day injuries and mishaps.

Emergency Index

What's involved in taking first aid?

A comprehensive course generally takes either a weekend or four or five week nights. Some teaching is done with books, videos, and/or lectures, but you also spend time trying out practical skills; this can be a lot of fun, especially if you take along a buddy to be your partner. A typical course covers the immediately life-threatening problems of choking, stopped breathing, and severe bleeding, and other topics such as burns, poisonings, cuts, broken bones, sprains, head injuries, and allergic shock. Some courses include CPR (cardiopulmonary resuscitation), but CPR is also taught separately.

 Isn't first aid mostly common sense?

While a lot of first aid seems like 'common sense' once you've learned it, untrained people can make serious mistakes because they don't understand

---

Cardiopulmonary resuscitation (CPR)

CPR is a simple technique for helping someone whose heart has stopped beating ('cardiac arrest'). It involves alternately 'pumping' the heart by pressing down on the chest, and giving mouth-to-mouth breathing. Although people often associate CPR with heart attacks, the most common situation in which it is used on children is respiratory arrest; that is, the child stops breathing and the heart soon stops beating as a result. A child may stop breathing for many reasons, including:

- choking

- asphyxiation (such as strangling, smoke inhalation, or getting a plastic bag caught over the face)

- near-drowning

- electric shock

- allergic shock (including food allergies and insect stings)

- poisoning (including drug or alcohol overdose)

- an epileptic convulsion

- a diabetic emergency

- a violent blow to the chest (in a fall or collision, for example)

CPR courses generally include first aid for choking and for stopped breathing, since the three conditions often go together. Techniques are slightly different for infants, children aged 1 to 8, and 'adults' over age eight; be sure the course you sign up for includes the age group you are most concerned about.

---

what's going on in the injured person, or what the first-aid priorities are. Sometimes what seems like the obvious first step is in fact very dangerous.

Besides, it's not easy to stop and think sensibly in an emergency. A good first-aid course does more than just teach you facts; it also drills you in a simple 'A B C' routine to help you handle a frightening situation in an organised, logical way. It should give you the confidence to stay calm yourself; to reassure the child; and to *take charge of the scene*, stopping other people from doing damage to the child.

Choking (Any Age)

If the baby or child can breathe or talk or cough, be reassuring but don't interfere; he or she will probably manage to cough up the obstruction. If you do an emergency manoeuvre on a child who doesn't really need it, you may do unnecessary damage.

If the baby or child can't breathe or talk or cough, or makes only a faint wheezing or whistling sound, follow the steps below. Note that if this isn't your own child, you must have the permission of whoever is in charge of the child. If no such person is present, you don't need permission unless the child is old enough to understand the risk and give 'informed consent.' After the obstruction is cleared, the child *must be checked by a doctor,* even if he or she seems fine; there is a slight chance that the life-saving manoeuvre may have caused internal bleeding.

The safe approach

In the event of an emergency:

S hout for help.

A pproach with care (protect yourself – e.g. in cases of electrocution or bleeding see page 210).

F ree from danger (remove child from danger).

E valuate (ask the child 'are you alright' and gently shake shoulders). If no response, call ambulance if possible and proceed with CPR.

Conscious Choking Baby (under Age One)

If anyone else is around, explain that the baby is choking and ask that an ambulance be called (dial 111).

Lay the baby face down on your forearm, cradling the face in your hand and pinning one leg between your arm and body. Tilt the baby slightly *head downward* so that gravity will help move the obstruction out.

Use the heel of your other hand to give five blows to the baby's shoulder-blade area. Adjust the force of the blows to the baby's size, to drive out the obstruction without doing unnecessary injury.

If the choking continues, roll the baby face up on your other forearm, holding the head securely in your hand. Again, tilt the baby slightly head downward. Imagine a line between the baby's nipples; line up your middle three fingers at this line, and then *lift* the top finger and use the other two fingers to thrust straight down five times.

If the choking continues, roll the baby back to the first arm and repeat the manoeuvres – five back blows, then five chest thrusts – until the obstruction is clear. If this is not successful give five attempts at rescue breathing then repeat five back blows and five chest thrusts.

The Heimlich manoeuvre

When we start to choke on something, we usually cough and clear the obstruction out of the way. We need help only if the blockage is so complete that we can't cough hard enough to get rid of it.

For the Heimlich manoeuvre to be most effective, the flat of the rescuer's fist should be between the victim's ribcage and navel, and each thrust should be as sudden and forceful as a cough. The sudden pressure forces air out of the lungs and, with luck, drives the obstruction out of the airway.

Conscious Choking Child (over Age One)

Stand or kneel behind the child, depending on the child's height. Make one hand into flat-sided fist, thumb outside. Place this fist just above the child's belly-button and cup your other hand over it (see diagram on page 208).

Now pull both hands upward and inward to imitate a forceful 'cough.' (The larger the child, the harder the motion should be.) If the first few thrusts don't clear the obstruction, continue the manoeuvre, making the thrusts harder. This is known as the 'Heimlich manoeuvre.'

Unconscious (Any Age)

If you can't awaken your child by pinching the earlobes, tapping the soles of the feet, and calling loudly in both ears, the child is likely unconscious. *Call an ambulance at once.* Dial 111.

Unless you suspect a head or spinal injury (see below), gently roll the child onto his or her back, tilt the head up slightly, and see if you can hear or feel breathing, or see the chest moving. If not, attempt five rescue breaths while you wait for the ambulance. Seal your mouth over the child's mouth or nose (if using mouth alone then pinch the nose closed using your thumb and index finger). If the child is breathing, gently roll the child face down on a flat surface, with the head turned to one side and the chin tilted slightly up; this will help keep the throat open and clear so the child can breathe.

If you do suspect a head or spinal injury, check the breathing as well as you can *without moving the child.* As long as the child is breathing, he or she should not be moved except by trained personnel.

Severe Bleeding

Apply pressure to the wound immediately, to stop the bleeding. Use your bare hand, or the child's bare hand, if necessary. It's essential to stop the loss of blood as quickly as possible.

For bleeding think RED

R = *rest* (to slow the pulse rate, which in turn slows the bleeding)
E = *elevation* (raising the wound above heart level slows the bleeding)
D = *direct pressure* (to stop the bleeding as quickly as possible)

Protecting yourself

If you are helping a bleeding child, there is a small chance you may be exposed to blood-borne diseases such as AIDS and hepatitis B. Be sure your first-aid kits have plenty of rubber or latex gloves. If no gloves are available, you must decide whether to risk the blood contact or not; if you decide to do so, wash thoroughly with soap and hot water as soon after as possible.

Once you have pressure on the wound, elevate the injured part above heart level, if that's practical and if the child's injuries permit. For example, if the child's foot is bleeding, lay the child down and prop the leg up on pillows. (A child who may have an injury to the neck or back should not be moved.)

Keep the child still, and be reassuring.

Find the cleanest dressing you can, and bandage the wound tightly enough to keep pressure on it, but not so tightly that you cut off circulation. *Do not* remove dressings, even if they get soaked with blood; just put new bandages over the top. *Do not* remove anything embedded in a cut, but be very careful not to bump the embedded object or to put pressure on it. Seek medical help at once.

Severe Burns

Cool the area immediately; a burn keeps on burning until the skin is cooled down. Applying water is usually the fastest method. Remove tight jewellery or clothing before swelling starts, but don't try to remove anything that's stuck to the burn. Do not apply creams or ointments, or any 'linty' dressing (such as facial tissue); special jelly-covered burn dressings are available in drugstores.

Burns are more serious in children, and have a high risk of infection. Any significant burn to a child should be checked by a doctor.

Poisoning

If there is an empty package or other evidence of the cause of poisoning, pick it up. *Call a poison control centre.* Check the front of your phone book for the number, or call the New Zealand National Poison's Centre: **03 474 7000**. *Do not* apply home remedies unless you are advised to do so by a poison control centre or a doctor.

Where to Find Support and Information

General Parenting

Barnardos

Helping children experience a cycle of success through effective care, support and education.

National Office
PO Box 6434, Wellington
Ph: 04 3857560
Fax: 04 382-6700
E-mail: information@
barnardos.org.nz
Website: www.barnardos.org.nz

Early Childhood Development / Nga Kaitaunaki Kohungahunga

A government agency supporting parenting and education of children 0 – 5 years.

PO Box 9951
Te Aro, Wellington
Ph: 04 381 9800, Fax: 04 381 9801
E-mail: info@ecd.govt.nz
Website: www.ecd.govt.nz

Your local office contact details are in your telephone book.

Family Information Service

Information is available on: medical conditions and treatment, disabilities, hospitalisation, parent support groups, coping with death and illness, parenting issues relating to children with health problems and disabilities.

Starship Children's Hospital
Private Bag 920 24
Level 3, Park Road
Grafton, Auckland
Ph: 09 307 4955
Fax: 09 307 4979
E-mail: SSFIS@ahsl.co.nz

Parent & Family Resource Centre Inc.

For help in finding: information, parent support groups, parent education and training resources, community services and resources, legal and advocacy services.

PO Box 13 385
Onehunga, Auckland
Ph: 09 636 0351
Fax: 09 636 0354

Parent to Parent New Zealand

A support and information network for parents of children with special needs.

National Office
PO Box 234
Waikato Mail Centre
Ph/fax: 07 834 1108
Or call toll-free on 0508 236 236 to find your nearest local group.
E-mail:
p2pnational@compuserve.com

Parenting with Confidence

An organisation running community-wide parenting seminars and providing resources for families.

PO Box 37 708
Parnell, Auckland
Ph: 09 307 0025
Fax: 09 307 0065
E-mail: pwc@parenting.org.nz
Website: www.parenting.org.nz

Royal New Zealand Plunket Society Inc.

Plunket operates a 24-hour information service for parents and caregivers: 0800 933 922
See your phonebook for your local office.

National Office
PO Box 1480, Dunedin North
Ph: 03 477 0110
Fax: 03 477 5164
Website: www.plunket.org.nz

Te Tari Puna Ora O Aotearoa/New Zealand Childcare Association

For the promotion and maintenance of high standards of education and care for young children.

PO Box 11 863
Manners Street, Wellington
Ph: 0064 4 3846947
Fax: 0064 4 3847149
Website: www.nzchildcare.ac.nz

Triple P Positive Parenting Programme

A parent education organisation offering seminars, information and training courses.

PO Box 74 025
Market Rd, Auckland
Ph: 09 520 7164
Fax: 09 520 0698
E-mail: triplep@xtra.co.nz

213

Allergy & Breathing Disorders

Allergy Awareness Association Inc.
PO Box 56 117
Dominion Rd, Auckland
Ph: 09 623 3912
Fax: 09 623 0091
E-mail: mail@allergy.org.nz

Asthma New Zealand
PO Box 67 066
Mt Eden, Auckland
Ph: 09 623 0236
Fax: 09 623 0774
E-mail: aas@asthma-nz.org.nz

Asthma and Respiratory Foundation NZ
National Office
PO Box 1459, Wellington
Ph: 04 499 4592
Fax: 04 499 4594
E-mail: arf@asthmanz.co.nz
Website: www.asthmanz.co.nz

Local asthma society contact details are in your phone book.

Behavioural Problems

ADDvocate
A nationwide umbrella organisation of support groups for parent/caregivers and teachers of children with ADD and ADHD.

Ph: 09 846 4128
E-mail: addburns@ihug.co.nz

ADHD Association Inc.
Resource Information Centre
652A Dominion Rd
Balmoral, Auckland
Ph: 09 623 5380
Fax: 09 623 4051

Breastfeeding

La Leche League NZ
PO Box 1270
Wellington
Ph/fax: 04 471 0690
E-mail: lllnz@clear.net.nz
Website: www.lalecheleague.org/LLLNZ

Local group contact details are in your phone book.

Burns

NZ Burn Support Charitable Trust Inc.
National Office
Dacre, RD 15
Invercargill
Ph: 03 231 3118

Colic Support Group
Contact: Fay Nunnerley
Ph: 09 410 0077
Fax: 09 410 4005
E-mail: Fay@ihug.co.nz

Cot Death

NZ Cot Death Association
National Office
597 Rosebank Road
PO Box 19 296
Avondale, Auckland
Ph: 09 828 5155
Fax: 09 828 3122

Maori SIDS Prevention Team
National Office
Maori Health Unit
Private Bag 92019, Auckland
Ph: 09 373 7599 ext. 7601
Fax: 09 373 7074

Pacific SIDS Prevents Programme
Pasifika Healthcare
199 Lincoln Road
Henderson, Auckland
Ph: 09 837 1780

OR Department of Maori and Pacific Health
University of Auckland
Healthcare Services
Private Bag 92019, Auckland
Ph: 09 373 7599 ext. 7601
Fax: 09 373 7074

Eating Disorders Association NZ
An Auckland based charity which offers support and information to anyone affected by eating disorders.

PO Box 80 142
Green Bay, Auckland

Ph: 09 818 9561
Fax: 09 818 9568
E-mail: anorexia@xtra.co.nz

Epilepsy New Zealand
National Office
PO Box 1074, Hamilton
E-mail: national@epilepsy.org.nz
Call toll-free on 0800 20 21 22 to contact your local branch
Website: www.epilepsy.org.nz

First Aid

Order of St. John
National Headquarters
PO Box 10 043, Wellington
Ph: 04 472 3600
Fax: 04 499 2320
E-mail: pceo@nhq.osj.org.nz
Website: www.stjohn.org.nz

Consult your phone book for your local office.

Kids Foundation
A not-for-profit organisation set up to support New Zealand children and adults diagnosed with Primary Immunodeficiencies (PIDs).

National Office
50 Omahu Rd
Remuera, Auckland
Ph: 09 523 5550
Fax: 09 523 5551
E-mail: kidsnz@nznet.gen.nz
Website: www.pidsnz.co.nz

215

national Kidney Foundation

PO Box 139, Christchurch
Ph: 03 379 1594
Fax: 03 365 2390
E-mail: kidney@cmrf.org.nz

Poisons

NZ National Poisons & Hazardous Chemicals Information Centre (NZNPHCIC)

School of Medicine
University of Otago
PO Box 913, Dunedin
Ph: (Urgent) 03 474 7000
Ph: (Non-urgent) 03 479 1200
Fax: 03 477 0509
E-mail: ntg@otago.ac.nz

Road Safety

Land Transport Safety Authority (LTSA)

Head Office
PO Box 2840, Wellington
Ph: 0800 699 000
Fax: 04 494 8601
Consult your phone book
for your regional office.

Safety

Child Safety Foundation

PO Box 56-313, Dominion Road
Mt Eden, Auckland
Ph: 09 638 7603 or
0800 CHILD SAFETY
Fax: 09 638 9357

Safekids Information Centre

PO Box 19-544
Avondale, Auckland
Ph: 09 820 1193
Fax: 09 820 1191
E-mail: safekids@iconz.co.nz
Website: www.safekids.org.nz

Injury Prevention Research Centre (IPRC)

Department of Community Health
University of Auckland
Private Bag 92019, Auckland
Ph: 09 373 7999 ext. 6348
Fax: 09 373 7503
Website: www.auckland.ac.nz/ipc

Injury Prevention Research Unit (IPRU)

Dept. of Social &
Preventive Medicine
University of Otago
PO Box 913, Dunedin
Ph: 03 479 8342
Fax: 03 479 8337
Website: www.otago.ac.nz/ipru

NZ Recreation Association

(For playground safety)
National Office
PO Box 13 396
Johnsonville, Wellington
Ph: 04 478 38314
Fax: 04 478 5237

Water Safety New Zealand
PO Box 10-126, Wellington
Ph: 04 801 9600
Fax: 04 801 9599
Ph: 09 309 4596 (toll free to
Wellington from Auckland)
Ph: 03 366 4718 (toll free to
Wellington from Christchurch)
E-mail: wsnz@watersafety.org.nz
Website: www.watersafety.org.nz

Index

Hair growth, 97
Haloperidol, 172–3
Head-banging, 92
Head injuries, and NLDs, 185
Headache, 196–8
  brain tumours, 196
  mumps, 159
  scarlet fever, 163
  tension, 197
  and vomiting, 71
  See also Migraine headache
Hearing problems, 110–11
Heartburn, and chest pain, 198
Heimlich manoeuvre, *209*
Helmets, bicycle, 134–5, *135*
Hepatitis, 81, 157–8
Hepatitis A, 157
Hepatitis B, 157–8
  immunisation, 25, 26, 28, 33
Herbal teas, 44
Heredity
  and abdominal pain, 191
  in ADHD, 178
  and conduct disorders, 172
  and learning disabilities, 185
Hirsutism, 97
Hives (urticaria), 98
Homatropine methylbromide, 43
Home births, 16–17
Hospital, discharge from, 21
Human herpes virus-6, 162
Hydrocephalus, and NLDs, 185
Hyperactivity, 166, 173, 176
Hyperkinesis, 176
Hypertrichosis, 97
Hypnotherapy,
  and bedwetting, 64
Hypothyroidism, 19

I
Ibuprofen, 52
  for sunburn, 101
Imipramine (Tofranil), 63
Immune response, 48
Immunisation, 25–8
  schedule, 26
  side effects of, 32–5
  teenagers, 34
  tetanus, 163
In-line skating injuries, 146
Infants
  bathing, 22
  car restraints, 130–2
  feeding, 113–19
  normal stool of, 72
  spilling, 67–8
  See also Breast-fed infant
Injuries
  and childhood, 128–49
  at home, 136–44
  and painful urination, 77
  playground, 146
  risk of, 129–30
  See also Falls
Intestinal infection,
  and vomiting, 70
Intussusception, 73
  and vomiting, 70–1
IQ tests, 185–6
Iron, 120, 122, 127
  supplements, 114
Isotretinoin (Accutane),
  acne, 102